PROUD FLESH

A MEMOIR OF MOTHERHOOD, INTIMATE VIOLENCE, AND RECLAIMING PLEASURE

CATHERINE SIMONE GRAY

North Atlantic Books
Huichin, unceded Ohlone land
Berkeley, California

Published by
North Atlantic Books
Huichin, unceded Ohlone land
Berkeley, California

Cover art and design by Amanda Weiss
Book design by Happenstance Type-O-Rama

Printed in Canada

Proud Flesh: A Memoir of Motherhood, Intimate Violence, and Reclaiming Pleasure is sponsored and published by North Atlantic Books, an educational nonprofit based in the unceded Ohlone land Huichin (Berkeley, CA) that collaborates with partners to develop cross-cultural perspectives; nurture holistic views of art, science, the humanities, and healing; and seed personal and global transformation by publishing work on the relationship of body, spirit, and nature.

To protect the privacy of real individuals and for the author's protection, some names and identifying details have been changed.

North Atlantic Books's publications are distributed to the US trade and internationally by Penguin Random House Publisher Services. For further information, visit our website at www.northatlanticbooks.com.

Library of Congress Cataloging-in-Publication Data
Names: Gray, Catherine Simone, author.
Title: Proud flesh : a memoir of motherhood, intimate violence, and reclaiming pleasure / Catherine Simone Gray.
Description: Huichin, unceded Ohlone land, Berkeley, California : North Atlantic Books, [2025] | Includes bibliographical references and index.
Identifiers: LCCN 2024034420 (print) | LCCN 2024034421 (ebook) | ISBN 9798889841265 (trade paperback) | ISBN 9798889841272 (ebook)
Subjects: LCSH: Gray, Catherine Simone. | Mothers--United States--Biography. | Sexual abuse victims--United States--Biography. | Motherhood--Psychological aspects. | Healing--Psychological aspects. | Mind and body. | Psychic trauma.
Classification: LCC HQ759 .G754 2025 (print) | LCC HQ759 (ebook) | DDC 306.874/3--dc23/eng/20241008
LC record available at https://lccn.loc.gov/2024034420
LC ebook record available at https://lccn.loc.gov/2024034421

1 2 3 4 5 6 7 8 9 FRIESENS 30 29 28 27 26 25

This book includes recycled material and material from well-managed forests. North Atlantic Books is committed to the protection of our environment. We print on recycled paper whenever possible and partner with printers who strive to use environmentally responsible practices.

For my mother
and my grandmothers

AUTHOR'S NOTE

When I began writing this book, I didn't want to tell you about the sexual violence, the emotional violence, and their legacy of intrusive thoughts and feelings in new motherhood. I wanted to tell you only about the pleasure and the healing that are possible on the other side. I wanted to protect you. I wanted to promise that it wouldn't be harrowing. I wanted to protect you the way a mother might want. Because she loves you.

I couldn't write it that way, though. It had no bones. That story couldn't walk us to a new place, you and me, the two of us together.

What I have instead is this: when I sit down to write to you, there is a sticky note on my desk that says, *May this work be for the highest good of all.* As you're reading, know that our highest good is the place where my eyes rest in between the keystrokes.

My oldest son, a second grader, asked me recently, *Why would you want to write about things that have already happened?* I smiled. I thought of his notebook where he draws fantasy creatures, some winged, some with fangs, some with both.

Before I could answer, he continued, *Would you rather write about the past or the future?*

Oh, my love, I write about the past so we can have a future.

But I tell him: *Writing about the past can help me figure out questions about myself and how I became who I am. I know that other people are trying to figure out things about themselves, too. We learn from each other by telling our true stories.*

A simple, bath-time answer. One answer.

I want you to be in tune with your highest good when you're reading, as only you know how. Take care of yourself first and close the book whenever you need to. Know that in these pages, the sun will come up over and over again. Even at midnight, the sun shines somewhere.

CONTENTS

proud flesh:
exuberant granulation tissue in a poorly healed wound,
characterized by florid, "geographic" scarring
on the skin surface

McGraw-Hill Concise Dictionary of Modern Medicine

PROLOGUE

Exactly ten years after I was raped, my vagina blossomed. It flowered from the place where I tore in childbirth, a garden of ruby red scar tissue. *Proud flesh*, I would later learn it was called. The biggest stalk was as long as my pinkie finger, from the tip to the last knuckle. My doctor handed me a mirror. "See that beefy red flap there? It bleeds when I touch it," she said, prodding the slug of tissue with a long Q-tip under a spotlight, illuminating my most private center. "Your body is actually overhealing."

I was four months postpartum from my second baby, and my vagina was still aching with heaviness. The places where I was stitched after birth felt like a tightly laced corset, a sharp saddle I rode all day. I leaked trickles of urine when I bent over or stood up from a chair, and my crotch felt barely held together, with my organs weighing heavier on the fault line of my perineum each hour.

Overhealing? That was a new one. *Healed, healing, have healed, will heal.* Healing had been the work of a decade since escaping the abusive relationship that had started when I was a month shy of seventeen.

With my backless clinic gown draped over me, Dr. S rubbed four six-inch-long wooden matchsticks of silver nitrate up my vagina to burn the ruby scar tissue. A metal vise and three hands stretched me open. With a mirror, I watched the tissue fizzle from red to gray, from blood to cinders.

After pulling off her tight blue gloves, Dr. S walked to my side and held out her hand to help me sit up. As we talked, my eyes squinted, and I nodded as a metallic nausea ballooned my head.

"The vagina is a very forgiving place—one of the most forgiving places on the body," she said. "It's designed to stretch and tear and return to a healthy state. It's basically made to withstand trauma."

Are all women made to withstand trauma? Designed to stretch and tear and return to a healthy state? Are women's bodies geographies of forgiveness? When I, mother of two, stood from my chair, my vagina became a heavy undertow, a drag below me. I couldn't do anything without being aware of it. Similarly, not a day goes by that I don't think about the man who raped me. An awareness in perpetuity.

I still lived in the city of Jackson, Mississippi, where for four and a half years, my first boyfriend had grown increasingly controlling, manipulative, and violent, escalating in rape weeks before I finally made my escape.

The blue house under the pines where I lived with my new little family of four was right around the corner from the gas station where J and I used to buy strawberry sodas in the summer, Pink Floyd drifting out the rolled-down windows of his white Corolla. Less than a mile from the hospital where my first baby was born was the apartment where J and I lived for three years. And the house where he raped me was right across the street from a playground where other moms invited me to meet them for playdates. There were geese there, a walking trail, and arches of lights during the holidays. My daily landscape was a geography of memory, with the violent ending always there. And somewhere in my city, in a parking lot or a coffee shop or a car next to me at the stoplight, he could be there, too. He could be anywhere I went, J and his penis.

In the six months after the scars in my vagina were found, I would undergo eight chemical burns to kill the extra scar tissue so that the original wound could heal.

In each session, my doctor colored my scars with silver nitrate. In the medical world, these were not serious treatments but minor events, in-office visits, not even called *procedures*. But for me, they were profound. Wounding and healing were at war at the center of my body, deep inside my caldera in a place no one could see.

This isn't what we have in mind when we say *healing*. Not burning our insides. Not killing living parts of ourselves. But I already knew that healing wasn't just lavender baths and light-dappled forest retreats.

What happens when survivors become mothers?

Write from the scars, not the wound, I've heard over and over in recent years. It sounds like a reasonable idea. We should let healing happen before we expose the vulnerable tissues to the world. Healing looks like: gaping, weeping, bleeding, crusting. A wound becomes a scab, a scab becomes a scar. Closure. Freedom.

But what happens when a scar becomes its own wound?

The first time my vagina was burned, I knew in an instant that something significant was happening. In the burning was a pathway.

I could wait forever to tell this story while the wound becomes a scar. The truth is that closure is only another beginning.

PART ONE

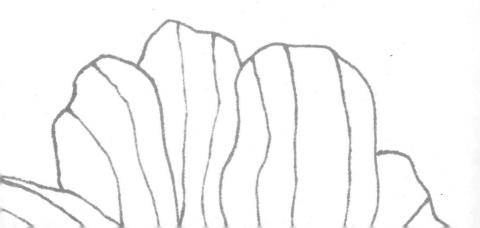

PINHOLE

I'd never seen myself naked before. Not like this. And neither had my husband.

In the photo he took, I am ten months pregnant, days away from giving birth to our first child. I sit naked and cross-legged on our back porch floor. My ripening breasts hang over my mountain of belly, and my chin bows down toward the drift of majestic overhang I have grown. My face vanishes in the dark slot canyon of my black hair. One areola shines straight forward, a massive brown radial on my breast, while the other one is obscured under falls of my loose curls. My right hand rests on my knee while my left disappears under the shadow of my belly, fading into pubic hair. Behind me, the eastern morning light lands on our backyard's twisted huckleberry branches. Before me, shadows. Grounded and solid, I look like a warrior readying for battle, but instead of holding a sword, I cradle my belly. Instead of armor, I am naked.

It was the first time I had asked Lloyd to take nude photos of me. I hardly ever let him see me fully naked. When I undressed for bed, I turned toward the closet as I unstrapped my bra or I emerged from the bathroom already wrapped in my nightgown. I hadn't always been like this. My freshman year of college, I posed for a local artist who painted on my bare skin with a geometry of seafoam green and then photographed me—collarbones, breasts, ribcage, mermaid hair. Two of those photos were even framed on our bedroom wall. But in the eleven years since, my body had shied back into itself, not for modesty but for self-containment.

Now I wanted to be seen again and wasn't afraid to be seen, every dimpled and curved inch of me highlighted by natural light. My pregnant belly emboldened me. Stretched to the limits of my skin to carry the next generation, I shape-shifted.

"Can the neighbors see me?" I asked Lloyd before I shed my covering. Our back porch is elevated several feet off the ground, and from that perch, I could see the backyards of the three adjacent houses over our wooden fence.

"Yes, I think so," he said, turning his head north to south, his focused eyes scanning the properties as if he were taking in a vista view.

It didn't stop me. I lowered myself onto my hands and knees and then leaned back onto my heels, pulling my nightgown over my head.

My first son was not born from my vagina. He was born from a six-inch incision above my pubic bone. The doctor dropped my placenta in a bin that said *MEDICAL WASTE*, and two days later, Lloyd drove us home while a summer thunderstorm gathered above us.

At my six-week postpartum checkup after the C-section, an assertive young nurse who bounced with forward momentum walked me to the hallway checkpoint where we always stopped for blood pressure, temperature, and weight. I shuffled behind her, my belly still a landslide that I felt could drop off if I moved too quickly.

"Are you having any postpartum?" she asked while I stepped on the scale, barely looking at me while she flipped through papers in a manila folder.

"Postpartum?" I asked. By definition, wasn't my whole existence now postpartum?

"Postpartum depression."

"Oh, um, no, I don't think so," I said. She'd asked me as casually as if inquiring what I had eaten for breakfast. She walked me to the exam room.

In pregnancy, I'd done all the things I thought a good mother did. I took three months of childbirth classes, washed gender-neutral baby clothes in unscented detergent, and curated a feminist board-book collection. I steadily tracked my baby's weekly growth from a blueberry to an avocado to a cantaloupe, meditating on whether I was building a spinal column, retinas, or vocal cords that week. With a cheery orange felt-tipped pen, I labeled index cards for the tiny garments in drawers that I marked like rows in a garden. *Footed pajamas, newborn to 3 months.* I interviewed three doctors and visited two out-of-state birth centers before deciding on a local doctor I trusted. I built my natural birth plan with the word processing template of a resumé and pasted a happy thumbnail of my husband and me, the young expectant parents, glimmering from the corner. I wanted to get a 4.0 in motherhood. *Mother cum laude.*

It wasn't just about accolades or checking boxes, though. Nothing was more important to me than being a good mother. If I could have given myself a superlative in the yearbook for freshman mother class of 2016, it would have been Most Likely to Succeed. There was my master's degree in curriculum and instruction, my years of babysitting and teaching kids from spit-up age to track-star age, and then there was my nature. The way I've always been. My whole life I've been called *a good listener, patient, diligent.* Nana Jojo says that from the time I was three years old, I always turned around to make sure that she was following behind me, checking on her like a mama duck.

But in the six weeks since becoming a mother, on a handful of midnights, I'd sat in my purple nursing chair Googling the symptoms of postpartum depression before closing the browser window, unsatisfied. I didn't feel hopeless, have dramatic mood swings, cry excessively, or have thoughts of harming myself or the baby. But I didn't feel the way I thought I would either. And there was that one time that we drove by a large body of water, and I imagined my baby falling out of my arms and sinking deeper and deeper into the brown-blue reservoir until I couldn't see his face anymore, and the despair I felt made me realize how much I couldn't bear to lose him. Did devotion count as love? Did wonder count as love? I was determined to love, and that felt like a good start. It was the best I could do. Hopefully it would be enough.

I wanted to be a mountain, unshakable. *Just be solid. Just be here.*

Here was a place I didn't recognize. My body was not the body I knew. Some nights I woke up with my breasts engorged with milk, like hard balloons full of sand. Other times they swung floppy like bags of icing. My lower body couldn't feel my hands when I touched it.

The doctor walked into the exam room. She sat down on a rolling stool, and we oohed and aahed over the baby.

"Let's take a look at the incision."

I lay back and rolled my underwear band down so that the doctor could see my cesarean scar. My pubic hair was growing back from the surgical shearing, low-lying black stubble like a putting lawn. The incision was not a painful searing at my center now, but the numb plot of skin between my belly button and pelvis made my womb feel distant, dead.

Nerves had been cut; they would regenerate, she explained. I nodded. Simple explanations for erasures of whole segments of my body.

The scar was red and fresh, barely crossed over from a wound. And one edge of it still lingered in wound territory. At the left edge of my incision, a lump of agitated scar tissue itched and bled. Every pair of underwear I owned had become stained with a circle of blood on the front, like one blooming polka dot. I'd been looking at it every day, checking for signs of infection. Pus, heat, fever. None.

The doctor leaned in closer and took a quick look at my pubic line.

"Ah, you have a pinhole," she told me almost cheerily. A small hole in the sutures that kept opening and reopening. *A pinhole.* She could seal it with a cauterizing chemical called silver nitrate. On this day, I let its name wash over me. She gloved up and held up a long wooden stick tipped with a silvery black sheen. With the tip she rubbed the pinhole near my pubic bone, and tingles of fire fingered my skin. My flesh stung and burned. It didn't make a sound, but in my mind, my wound crackled and sizzled, like oxygen escaping a log on the hearth.

Lloyd had gone back to work after two weeks, my mom had flown back to California, and my mother-in-law's stay had come to an end, too. Now I was alone in the house with my baby. I sat in the purple nursing chair that Nana Jojo had gifted for my baby shower.

Guider was so beautiful that he looked like a magical being. His black hair was as soft as the inside of a silky midnight corn husk. His eyes were broad and knowing, like dark seed pods. His upper lip hung over his lower lip, giving him a serious, owl-like countenance. His long monkey feet tried to wrap around my finger. Like a moonflower, he had grown in my darkness. *My* baby. I said it to myself in equal parts awe and disbelief, waiting for the truth of it to sink in. Awe flitted around me, light as a hummingbird. He came from my body—amazing. But another thing flitted, wingless, darting from shadow line to shadow line like a lizard. It had been restless in me since birth.

I had imagined my baby's face every day I carried him, sculpted it a thousand ways. I thought that I would recognize him right away, a face I had known for all time, his features like coordinates mapped deep in my psyche. *This is my flesh and blood.* But when I looked at him, I didn't detect Lloyd or me; I saw someone entirely new. A stranger.

Until one morning I looked down at Guider, and I saw my ex-boyfriend's face. My ex-boyfriend, my abuser, my rapist. I wasn't even sure what to call him anymore. I didn't want him to be *my* anything. For years I'd avoided saying J's name whenever possible to Lloyd. Sometimes I'd allude to *the past* or *the trauma* or explain, *because of where I've been*, which was code for: *life with J.* But it was a Voldemort situation. He Who Shall Not Be Named. As if merely saying J's name could give him power that would animate him and amplify his force in my life. At the same time, not needing to use his name was chilling, as if he were an omnipresent force, a capital h *He*, like God.

Lloyd and I had built a beautiful life together over our seven years, with fog machine Halloween parties and church book clubs on our back porch. Once our first baby was born, our community of love organized a Meal Train, with friends and family delivering us cashew noodles, cornbread, and collard greens. The mention of J, whether I used his name or not, always stung like a lack of gratitude for the life we'd built, as if no amount of goodness around me would be enough to move past the harm.

Yet, there was J's face on my baby. His eyes, his lips. On my baby. As if Guider were his baby. My heart beat faster. Shock and revulsion pounded.

Many times before I'd thought about how narrowly I had escaped a lifetime of being connected to J through a shared child. How lucky I was to be truly free. I'd even imagined the arguments we would have had trying to co-parent, the bang-'em-up movies he'd want to show our kid that I didn't find appropriate. I imagined J pulling up in my driveway, giving our child a fist bump, and buckling him into the back seat for the weekend while I stood awkwardly to the side, waving goodbye with a peach pit in my gut. My kid would come home smelling like cigarettes even though I'd made J promise not to smoke around our son.

But it wasn't true, I reminded myself. I'd been able to make a clean breakaway from J, and nothing had to connect us now. I didn't have to talk to him ever again. I certainly didn't have to parent with him. Guider never needed to know that name and that face. I breathed in and sucked the nothing deep below my breastbone. I kissed the top of my baby's head.

As I rocked Guider and stared out the window at the oak leaves that were shot through with light, I thought of a conversation with Lloyd a few weeks before, on our first walk as parents.

"Do you feel a strong connection to the baby, an overpowering love?" I had asked Lloyd. I felt safe amid the hundred-year perspective of the pines that towered over us. I wouldn't have been able to ask it inside the house: it would have filled the whole room; it would have busted the walls. Outside, though, it was like picking up a rough stone that could travel in my palm for a few paces before I set it down again.

"Not really. Not yet," Lloyd said with a calm steadiness. I looked up at the overcast sky, a balm of clouds above the treetops.

"Me either."

It felt natural for a father to need time to bond with his baby. But a mother's love? I thought it would rush into me as if the air had a new saturation of oxygen. Is there anything we expect to be more natural and powerful than a mother's love? I felt a gaping void where I expected the love to be. In awe that this beautiful tiny human came from me, committed to protecting him and to helping him thrive, but where was the eruption of love? My baby and I had recently been one rolling body; but since birth, I felt our separateness, like two pinballs dropping.

I couldn't verbalize it yet, but a crater of fear scooped wholeness from my center, like the blasted core of a mountain. *What if the abuse broke my ability to love with that depth? What if I'll always be less able to give and receive love because of the way I was violated?* It had been my deep fear for a long time that J had gotten the best of my love, the unfiltered and unguarded love that I hurled into the world before I knew how to stay safe. *No. He doesn't get to be here*, I asserted. Not with my son, not on our first walk as a family, not in this life I'm building. The relief reached me at a head level, but there was still something legless wriggling in my belly, like mosquito larvae.

My dreams of breastfeeding had been expressions of pastoral bliss, mother in a flowy white dress in a field of sunflowers. What I now had was the word *latch*. How a baby's mouth attaches to a nipple and areola. But also: *A metal bar with a catch and lever used for fastening a door or gate. To lay hold with, as if with the hands or arms.* It perhaps originates from the Greek *lambanein*, meaning *to take or seize*. Breastfeeding began as a physical struggle that required a whole team of hands. I sat topless in the purple nursing chair. Mom stood on my right side to keep the baby from pushing away off my breastbone, while Lloyd guarded my left side to keep Guider's feet from kicking my bruised cesarean incision.

I tried to rush my sandwiched breast into his mouth before his jaws clamped down on my nipples. The trick was to get him to open his howling mouth wide enough to get my breast inside, but our timing was out of sync, and his mouth chomped down a half-beat too soon in a shallow latch. When his mouth finally attached to my breast, a piercing pressure gripped me by the nipple and pulled, sharp as glass being ground into my breast. My toes curled. I tried to breathe in and relax my shoulders, but I braced against the pain. 1 2 3 4 5 6. If the sharp pressure didn't lessen by the time I got to 30, I promised myself that I would slip my finger in his cheek to detach him. 28 29 30. I wedged my finger between his gums like a fishhook, and he opened his mouth, searching for me, frantic. But his mouth wasn't open wide enough for my breast; it was going to clench my nipple again. I pulled back, afraid. He grunted an early cry, and that cry pried his mouth open wider. I used that gaping moment to stuff my breast in his mouth swiftly, and he chomped and pulled me in. This was our third try, so I tolerated the pain. His small body felt like a tense and desperate animal, the frenzy of hunger. In order to meet his hunger, I disappeared to somewhere outside my flesh, but I worried that he could sense he had an absent mother.

After fifteen minutes, his eyes began to soften, fluttering his lashes toward sleep. I was relieved that it was over, the feed successful. At the same time, watching him drift away into the bliss of himself on the numb edge of my body felt disconcerting. My nipples came out of his mouth white like plaster and crushed to a point like a flathead screwdriver. Bad latch.

Feeding time was every two hours. It sounds like a Sea World attraction—my body providing silvery, scaled handfuls of chum. I dreaded the next cycle, but whether or not my body liked it was irrelevant to me. Something was beginning to rumble in me, old stories like, *Love's not easy. This is what it takes.* Those stories had led me down dangerous paths with my body before, and I could feel that danger quaking inside me, the slippery clamp of love that takes so much.

Purple nursing chair. Haze of a winter sky out the window, branches naked. I was nursing Guider before nap time, and suddenly it was as if there were two of us in my body. There I was, the twenty-eight-year-old woman who wanted to be *a mama bear*, with lines of stretch marks and a six-inch scar on her belly. And then there was the seventeen-year-old girl having her nipples kissed in her boyfriend's bedroom. She appeared like a ghost when I lifted Guider to burp him, and he spit a curdled jelly mass on my neck that slid down between my breasts, past my belly button, and all the way to my underwear. The warm slickness of the fluid brought J's voice back.

You want me to cum on your face? Tell me, say it.

And me: *Cum on my face.*

I didn't remember the moment as a moving image so much as I smelled it: the semen and the spit-up. Something sharp and fermented from inside someone else's body that I wiped off my skin with a rag. My eyes got sticky and stung. I could have mopped the floor with my cheek and said I liked it, that's how low I suddenly felt, as if a giant hand had pushed me down.

I did sexy things. Your mother did sexy, dirty things even when she didn't like it, I could hear myself confessing in my head as my baby drifted into sleep on my chest, skin-to-skin. The heat of tears began to prickle me as we rocked. I wished I had another body to feed my child with and to press him against, one that hadn't been in that bedroom with J. Intellectually, I could see what was happening, internalization of the old Madonna–whore complex, which polarizes women between sacred or profane, whole or fallen, mothers or sexual. But even though I could diagnose it, I felt myself swept up in its current. Tumbled over by the intersection of the smells and the square footage of my flesh and the sweat slicking between my baby's skin and my breasts, I had the sense that when the Madonna was born, the whore came knocking. I thought I'd made peace with her. No name-calling or victim blaming here. I did what I needed to do to survive. My head insisted that I knew these things.

And yet bodies are what exist before stories and after stories. Bodies rush in to fill the gaps that our stories leave behind. My favorite poet Louise Glück writes: "We look at the world once, in childhood. / The rest is memory." Maybe I had known my body once, with J.

For the first months of my son's life, I tried to stack the memories of those years into an airtight sixty-gallon plastic bin, drive it through stoplight after stoplight to the city limits, shove it into a storage unit, slam the rolling metal door down to the concrete, lock the padlock, and drive away. Gone, never happened. I could walk back into my house and be the mother and wife I always imagined I would be. In this life, the big question of the morning was whether to attend the 9:30 or the 11:00 preschool storytime at the library, and all I needed to track was my baby's milestones, not how close my memories were.

In this life, J had never touched me—not when it felt exciting, not when it felt degrading—and we'd never told each other *I love you* or traced each other's freckles. We'd never joked about our make-believe future kids Uma and Boogar, and he'd never drawn us as a cartoon family, both of us bespectacled parents with lumps of wavy, mashed potato-mound hair, goofy grins. In this life, the first man who'd spooned me wouldn't go on to rape me.

Over dinner, as I spooned peas onto Guider's highchair tray, Lloyd said, "I think you're going to want to check out what

I saw today—it's a room full of vaginas." His eyes widened and stayed there for a few moments like a revelation. Lloyd was working at our alma mater as a grant writer and had stumbled upon the student exhibit while meeting with art professors. That week, I strapped Guider into his car seat and drove the five miles to campus. It was spring, and the azaleas were flaming. I pushed the stroller into a room as small as a walk-in closet. A line of vulvas bordered the walls on every side. Clay was shaped into genital folds on small square canvases and painted in shades of pink and brown. I counted them: twenty-five. I knew to call them *vulvas*, but I suspect that many others who'd passed the space had called them *vaginas* like Lloyd had or some cutesy name with a giggle attached. Among these vulvas, some had blood trickling down, some had brown hair pulled from costume wigs, and some had black-handled steak knives jammed into the vaginal opening.

I walked over to the artist's statement on the wall and read the name of the exhibit: *Violations . . . And Then I Became Angry*. My eyes shot down to the gallery note:

The work in this exhibition explores how frequently sexual assault occurs around us . . . I am interested in how violent acts reduce the human body to single body parts as their identity, as rape consumes victims' psyche and self-worth.

My heart began beating faster, the quickening of ideas. *How violent acts reduce the human body to single body parts as their identity.* I walked closer to one vulva until I was little more than a tongue's distance away. It was almost cartoonish in dimensions as it rose from the square. I turned around and did a quick scan of the room. Every three or four vulvas had a steak knife sticking out of the center, just like the statistic of sexual violence. The steak knives were impossible to look beyond; they demanded attention, unlike the invisible wounds we carry.

I walked closer to a brown vagina with a knife slicing from its center, and it was almost too painful to look at directly, the violence frozen in time. Not only was the vulva isolated from the rest of the body, literally disembodied, but there was no hand holding the knife either. It was as if the knife had always belonged there, just like the hair and the menstrual blood. The knife stayed there, forever, while whoever put it there walked out of the room and assimilated into the city around us.

In the background rose the sound of table saws and college laughter in the art studio next door. Guider began twisting against his stroller straps, grunting and blowing air through his left hand like a trumpet. Soon his grunts would escalate into cries. I walked back to the stroller and moved him toward the threshold. I lingered there, turning to take one last look at the room of vulva violations.

As I walked back to the car, across sidewalks I knew well from my college years, I thought of another wall I'd heard of on this campus: a wall of men. Years earlier, a friend who had also escaped an abusive relationship told me that when she stopped by the security office of our college campus at the end of senior year, she witnessed a collage of pictures on the wall—all photographs of men. The photo I'd provided of J was staring at her, along with the boyfriend of another friend we'd hardly seen since freshman year. These were all men who were banned from entry on campus. A whole wall of men.

Where are those other girls now? I'd wondered over the years. *Were they safe? Were they happy? Were they mothers having the same kinds of thoughts that I was?* There was always another presence that haunted me, too: all the women who haven't escaped.

It was after this day, after the vulva room, that my vagina began to speak to me. Not in words, but in sensations. I was in the bathtub when I first noticed the urge to push something out of my vagina. Across days, the urge persisted, incomprehensibly. I wanted something big to press me from the inside out, not an object but something that was mine. I don't think I'd ever noticed a feeling in my vagina before, except for the occasional pulse of desire or an itch of infection. My vagina had been a quiet, empty place. Hidden. Now it had a need I didn't understand. I had no name for this need. I stood in the bathroom alone trying to make sense of it while Lloyd changed Guider's diaper.

There was no mistaking it: My vagina wanted not to receive inward but to expel outward. To push. To exert force. As strong as any sexual desire, this was what I imagined the urge to penetrate might feel like, a sleeping hardness of my own ready to awaken.

But it would still be one year and six months before my vagina tore in childbirth when my second son was born. Even longer before I could understand what this wound needed to tell me.

mosquito

I am the one the mosquitoes find. In a July dusk, mine is the blood that gets siphoned. While other people can sit right next to me not getting a single bite, I am plumped up with a dozen welts on my legs in five minutes. My skin gives off a chemical that says, *Land here. I have the blood that will feed you.* From a young age, there were other hungers I'd attracted: people with longing and thwarted dreams; people with depression, disorders, and serial misfortune. People brought their heartaches and their secrets to me as if I was their new moon. By high school, I was a bright treasury of old wounds. When people call a sixteen-year-old *an old soul*, it means her blood is rich with nutrients and her skin is more invitation than barrier. It means people will come hungry. It means she has learned to feed them.

I called myself the love child of Joni Mitchell and Bob Marley. I called myself a flower child. My two braids each hung thick like a horse's mane almost to my hips, and my principal recited lines from "The Song of Hiawatha" when we passed in the hall. *See the face of Laughing Water / Peeping from behind the curtain.* Boys in my creative writing class called me Yoko. Tenor boys in chamber choir called me The Girl from Ipanema. I smiled, ready to be moonlight, starlight, firelight, sunshine, waterfall. After I watched a Woodstock documentary, my daydreams became expressions of naked bodies walking out of creek beds, long-haired people swaying to guitar music and kissing in fields. I wanted nothing more than to be there, in the middle of it, free. I was less interested in how it might feel when naked bodies touched than in being seen and known for all that I was.

In my bedroom, I looked at myself shirtless in the mirror and ran my hands along my breasts. They curved like plums at the bottom, and my areolas hung like iconographic halos. I did not look at myself as myself. I looked the way I imagined a boy would for the first time, discovering.

In the end, the first time someone saw me naked, he was a man, not a boy.

Mississippi in the summer is life gratified. Wild, teeming, dangerous, fraught. I grew up in a kingdom of mosquitoes, fire ants, hissing possums, and ripe blackberries burning in the sun. Mississippi in the summer is thick and amniotic, a heavy womb. Mosquitoes can spawn in as little as a bottle cap of rainwater, larvae twisting and wriggling into wings. Everything wants to come into existence, to be born, to have its chance to nurse on the land and to bleed.

I don't remember a first date with J, only that soon after we met at his band's show at The Mad Hatter in July, his CDs were stacked in my passenger seat. In my bedroom at my mom's house, he introduced me to Pink Floyd's *Wish You Were Here*. We passed a whole afternoon listening to the album and studying each other, with him pointing out the chord progressions with a tilt of his head and his finger in the air tapping the mastery of a sprawling, sparse guitar solo. His face looked almost pained at the most beautiful sections as he bit the inside of his lip.

I was not yet seventeen, with my head full of college essays and standardized test strategies, and he was twenty-four, with rent and a pay stub. He was smart, so smart that he knew college was a waste of time and that GPAs didn't count for much in life. He worked in the kitchen of a pub and smoked a pack of Winstons each day, spending the leftovers of his paycheck on video games and restaurant queso. The farthest from Mississippi he'd traveled was five hundred miles to the Smoky Mountains of Tennessee, while I'd already lived in four regions of the country and traveled to France six times to stay with my mother's family. He was the son of a barber, with little extra to go around, and my dad was a dual-specialist doctor who didn't notice if I charged band T-shirts and anti-war pins to his credit card.

"I'm just a simple man," he confessed in his cloudy Southern accent. "Do you think I'm a redneck? Why is someone like you interested in me?"

The thing is, as a fifth grader, I'd watched *Titanic* thirteen times in the movie theater. I marinated in the romance of Jack and Rose, the poor but spirited artist from steerage and the miserable rich girl trapped in a dull life of manners. The most enthralling love stories always seemed to have this forbidden quality: the star-crossed lovers and the trysts across the railroad tracks.

I did not feel I was a child; I was one year younger than my mother was when she became a mother. Besides, the boys in high school seemed young, their bodies spindly and awkward, their advances apologetic. They were not for me. With a tiny Christian high school class of sixty-two students, I felt more like a sister toward my classmates than a potential girlfriend or romantic partner. The guys walked me through calculus problems, and I walked them through their shy feelings and crushes.

I smelled like soap that came from a spring-green box, mixed with tobacco smoke and French fry oil. His forearms were creamy and muscular, shaped by thousands of hours of fingering the chords of bluegrass hollows. His hands were soft and thick, his nails trim and clean, his fingers confident. When he pressed his lips against my neck, he inhaled deeply.

When his soft lips pressed against mine, his tongue barely dipped into my mouth, as if we were peeking into each other. Up until now, kissing had been a one-off. I'd never had a boyfriend to practice kissing with, and so I'd never been able to move past that first slug-tongue awkwardness. J kissed me as if I was someone precious and good, like an intact shell he found before the ocean shattered it. This seemed important to him. The rest of the world disappointed him, but finally he'd found something perfect. I never wanted to be the reason he rolled his eyes.

I didn't know how lonely I had been, even in the middle of summer, even in a pile of my friends' heartbeats and laughing bellies. But suddenly it felt like opening the door of my car in winter, the interior holding a rush of hot air from the sun.

J's house was a rental near downtown, on a street with roofs withering to a point of near collapse. The House of Song had white paint that curled and peeled by the front door. When I walked in, J's dachshund, Red, named after the Willie Nelson album *Red Headed Stranger*, ran up to me and flopped onto

her back at my feet like a Vardaman sweet potato. She whim-
pered as she revealed the velvet skin on her belly. I leaned
down to rub her softness. I took it as a sign that his dog liked
me instantly. I was sure he noticed.

Inside, foam egg crate covered the walls in the band
room that were wallpapered with album covers, iconic vintage posters, and yellowing magazine cartoons. Guatemalan
blankets hung in the windows as curtains. Blond baby dolls
littered the carpet in sex positions, and dirty *Mario Bros.*
T-shirts and cargo pants gathered in piles.

I asked to use the bathroom, and J motioned for me to
take a right past the kitchen. The bathroom sink was fringed
with pilings of beard hair, rings of water, and saliva rust.
The toilet was worse. Somehow this was exciting to me, not
alarming, its sheer novelty, a marvel. Men live here. Men pee
here.

J lived with the drummer and the bassist of his band, and
the house felt like an orgy, not for sexual penetration but
for music. We sat in the living room on the sunken couch. J
grabbed a guitar that was leaning against the wall, and David
grabbed the upright bass that looked like it had been swiped
from a mariachi band. They talked about a Hitchcock movie
and then some Tom Waits banter, with a dingleberry poop
joke mixed in. It was hard to tell where the conversation
ended and the music began. They strummed and plucked
for a few measures as they spoke and then, minds synchro-
nized, they let the song take off. I admired the intimacy of
their wavelengths. Their band was becoming wildly popular
in Jackson, blending jazz, soul, rock, and reggae. They could
get a whole room on their feet.

Here, in the living room, I began to sing along to a chorus
I knew.

J kept an old Gatorade bottle in his bedroom that was full of water and a black cloud of dead fleas that he had picked off Red's belly, a macabre snow globe of parasites. As we talked, he searched Red's underside and added flea after flea to the bottle. She stayed still, quivering, a sweet little spud.

That night, he began to tell me everything. His brother's alcoholism and his father's cancer. His constant fear of death and his panic attacks. He shared his deep regret from boyhood for throwing a turtle into a cement ravine at the prompting of his friends. He told me about the dog collar he hung on his wall after his childhood pup died. He told me he was an insomniac; he couldn't sleep because he couldn't stop hearing the natural rhythm around him, a pattern for the dog barking next door and the whirring fan. Sometimes he stayed awake until 6 a.m. counting out measures of sound. He said he felt stupid telling me. I told him that I understood, and I listened with my full attention because I knew that it's not every day a shy boy feels safe to open up like this. I listened because he was showing himself to me, and that meant I could show myself to him, too.

And I began to tell him everything. The glacial crumbling of my parents' marriage in middle school, and the way they tug-of-warred me between them. How I missed my mom when she was away as a flight attendant, and I acted like I needed her less than I actually did because I didn't want her to feel bad for being gone half the time. The years I starved myself and how my parents didn't even notice. How I would have loved to have been visible enough to be sent to therapy or rehab like my friends. The way lying was my second fluent language because my dad thought everything was dangerous but I wanted to really live.

Soon I was at the House of Song every day. Other musicians and artists passed through as if it were a train stop on the City of New Orleans. I never knew who would be stopping by—an elegant jazz singer with vintage dresses and long, fiery hair, an old-time fiddle player with a twang, an experimental sketch performance artist who carried a keyboard under his arm? *This is the place.* I was in the middle of it. And soon I didn't even need to knock on the door to enter. I came in through the back door, where the boys kissed me on the cheek with a *Hey, sweetheart.*

J's favorite part of my body was the divot above my lips, the size of his pinkie's fingerprint. I thought it was sweet, that in the whole expanse of my wildflower body, he was attracted to a spot above my lip.

"You are the most beautiful person I've ever seen," he affirmed. I believed him. And it felt as if my life was finally beginning.

When my family moved to Mississippi when I was in sixth grade, I became aware of my difference in a way that I had never noticed before. Maybe it was a matter of being twelve years old and entering a new level of consciousness. Maybe it was because I was ethnically ambiguous and lacked language for my layers of identity. Maybe it was because my family hadn't lived in Mississippi for generations or in this country, for that matter. I was a first-generation American on Mom's side.

When I arrived at my fancy new private school, my teachers and my classmates' parents were always trying to connect me to someone they knew. *Do you have family in Gluckstadt?* they'd ask when they heard my German last name. They wanted to map blood coordinates of my kin and relate me to a person from the neighboring town. *Where do you go to church?* they tried next. *We don't really go to church*, I had to confess. Being an outsider felt rude because I offered no built-in reassurances that they could make sense of me. I learned to enunciate every syllable of my dad's specialty, *he-mat-o-path-ol-o-gy*, and the name of the hospital where he worked.

The pretty white girls in my class had silky, shiny hair that looked like it had been spun by angels overnight, while I had a frizzy bob of wires. When my sixth-grade science teacher asked us to pull a hair out of our heads to look at under the microscope, I panicked. I pulled one out from the front where my hair was finest, and I rubbed my finger over that blade of hair behind my back over and over, hoping I could make it something less like my own.

When my mom and I traveled, which was often since she was a flight attendant, strangers on planes would ask us where we were from. People raised their eyebrows at the mention of Mississippi—racism, miseducation, poverty, politics. I told the story like this: *Well, I live in Mississippi, but I was born in Florida and lived in New Hampshire and Iowa, and my mom is French.* I lived in Mississippi like it was a temporary state of being, like an anchor tattoo you press onto your skin only because it will wash off two days later. Mississippi was just where I happened to sleep, a place that had nothing to do with me, and I had nothing to do with her either.

J knew all the hidden spots around Jackson. The summer we met, we became explorers of remote train tracks, levees, creek beds, and trails. We drove through the western and southern half of the city that my dad had called unsafe. J wasn't afraid. He wasn't afraid of men with baggy clothes and paper bag tallboys who talked to the sky, and he didn't reach over to lock the doors. We kept the windows down, and he knew the names of the homeless men who rifled through trash cans; he pointed them out to me as we drove.

Maybe Mississippi was only rich-girl-private-school-weed-party boring. I could feel the place changing before my eyes, becoming known, becoming extraordinary. I could hear Mississippi like my mother starting to ask me, *Are you hungry, sweetie? I can make you something.*

"There's so many fish in the sea, Catherine. Just reel 'em in, play with them for a bit, and throw 'em back, throw 'em back," my aunt Deborah said while we sat on the back porch drinking lime margaritas we'd scooped from a bucket in our freezer. I lived with my mother and grandmother, and my aunt's presence on the weekend made it feel like a matriarchal sanctuary. My French nana scoffed at America's drinking laws, and in our house, I felt like an equal among women.

I laughed at Deb and shook my head. I knew these lines.

I'd watched so many of my mother's, aunt's, and grandma's romances go man-sour that I didn't expect much from men. I'd watched *I love you* turn into *Fuck you* and back again. This one flies a plane. This one is generous and buys diamonds. This one is cheap as hell but takes her to doctor's appointments. This one once played Big Bird on *Sesame Street*. This one plays the guitar and loves *Dances with Wolves*. I got tired of learning the men and of holding the bond that was gone just when I thought I could trust it. This one gave ultimatums. This one faked his own death. This one couldn't get his dick hard. This one wants her back; he can't live without her.

"Don't ever change your plans for a man," Nana said in her strong accent, taking a drag of her cigarette with a distinctly

French flair. "I know you, sweetie. You like to take care of every animal that's hurt. Since you were a little girl you were like that. Look—every mosquito bites you because you're so sweet." She clucked her tongue against her teeth and swatted my arm. "You're my strawberry girl, my little strawberry girl."

Another mosquito landed on me. I brushed it away, but it was already full of my blood.

"When I'm with you, I don't care about anything else," I confessed while I stroked J's hair. We sat like two noodles looped around each other in my papasan chair. "I forget about everything I need to do, and I don't know if that's a good thing. I make you late for band practices, late for work."

"As long as I have you, I don't need music or money or anything," he said. "Nothing else matters if I have you." He ran one finger over my eyebrow.

"Why do you love me?" I asked.

"Because of your boobs," he said, deadpan.

"Be serious."

"I am."

In my bedroom J made cryptic notes for me, prismatic drawings and word puzzles. He handed me this one:

Dear Catherine,
  __Y T__I__ T__ __E N__ __ __ T __ EA__ , __I__ __ __E
__E __A__IN__ G__O__ __ __E F__ __ __ __ __ E R?

It was my job to decode it. I found this message:

Dear Catherine,
  By this time next year, will we be saying goodbye forever?

It was no secret that I was leaving for college the next year. California or Portland already had my promise of a future. I was meant for a future far away from the bald cypress swamps and J's House of Song. I was promised to that future. But that promise was beginning to swell and warp, like wood outside in a Mississippi summer. The promise of a different future was beginning to circle around me. A little house. Yes, a little white house in Belhaven with wood floors, morning sunlight through the windows, a hammock on the front porch, and a garden on the side. We could have a few kids with my dark hair, his blue eyes; my poetry, his music. My daydreams became expressions of magnolia petals and baking pecan pies. I became aware of the urge to pull a blanket around him when he was cold.

You're supposed to be breaking away from this feeling, I told myself. Mom, Jojo, and Deborah had told me all their stories so that I could break away from this tired story: a lady taking care of her man, giving up everything for her man. I was the one daughter, the one granddaughter, the one niece. I was the one raised to break through that story.

J drew a cartoon portrait of me, but instead of a head, he gave me a cloud of ascending loops and swirls. I ended somewhere off the page, somewhere in his imagination.

Summer was ending. The heat doesn't give up willingly in Mississippi. One day it feels like high summer and then sometime in October, you wake up and feel a change. The heat reluctantly loosened its grip, not in one clean release but in sporadic gasps of relief. I invited J to my homecoming dance right as the mosquitoes began dying.

He showed up late to pick me up. He'd washed his hair, but I was so used to seeing his curls matted and dirty that he looked unlike himself, artificial and gelled. He'd missed shaving patches on his neck, and other spots reddened with razor burn. He was wearing his dad's brandy leather jacket and his collared date shirt, the white one with the beige stripes. He'd made an effort. But something felt off. What was it? Something wriggled in my gut. When he leaned in to hug, I left a gap.

Mom snapped pictures of us by the brick fireplace, and only when I flipped through them on my camera did I know: our bodies looked wrong next to each other. I looked young, and he looked old. I looked beautiful, and he looked run-down. My eyes sparkled and connected. His: flat and unreachable.

I stayed silent during most of the ride to the dance. I said I was mad that he was late, but I was more disturbed by the distance between us that I couldn't unsee. The promise of my future, the glimmer of my youth. The full lint drawer of his dreams, the beginning of a body touched by age, cynicism, and lack of self-care. But my tinge of repulsion was colored in by my guilt; he was self-conscious about his body, and working in the kitchen didn't leave him the money to outfit himself like the boys at school dressed by their doctor parents.

When we arrived, I was glad for the low lights of the dance outside under strands of white lights. J didn't want to dance; he was above it. He made his *Beavis and Butt-Head* face while he gyrated and then sulked in the corner. He hated high school. He made fun of my people, unforgivably privileged, in his eyes, and sang "Rich Girl" out the side of his mouth. There was no way for me to stand with a foot in both worlds: his world and the world of my friends. We left the dance early and went back to the House of Song. I felt too beautiful and hopeful to have such a disappointing night. My breasts would never be more perfect, and I'd trimmed my pubic hair that morning.

It was the year my best friends were getting their first serious boyfriends and losing their virginity. I decided that childhood was over, and my virginity was like a tidy y-axis I could draw between negative space and the positive infinity that awaited. I had the power to draw that line, and it was more power than I'd ever had with a man before, where I wasn't even allowed to have an opinion about George Bush at Dad's dinner table. I knew no way to become a woman faster than to have a man fucking me, and J was the man who squeezed my hand three times to say *I love you*, just like I had told him my papa used to do. Besides, I didn't like the distance that landed between us that night. I wanted to move through the gaping hole of that sadness and travel finally to a naked field with someone, free.

In his bedroom, I pulled my mom's black dress over my head.

"I'm ready."

"I'll go slow," he said. "Tell me if it hurts too much."

A SECOND-DEGREE WOUND

It's one of the scariest things I can imagine: my vagina tearing toward my anus, ripping like a sheet of Valentine construction paper.

But I don't feel my vagina tear when my second baby slips out of my body. I am bowed on all fours in my bedroom. The upper half of my body hangs limp over a green exercise ball, and my head bows toward my closet, the white crepe curtain close enough that my sweat drips onto it. I took such care in curating this birth room, with a crown of flowers high on the wall and a rainbow watercolor by the bed that says, *This is a new birth*, but now I can only stare at the same three square inches of waffle-weave until my entire world is compressed into that textured perimeter. My entire being hunches into a surrender to blood, breath, and heartbeat.

"Catherine, it's the first real fall morning out there," my photographer friend Jess says in a firefly-gentle voice between my contractions. I know what she's doing: she's reminding me that this labor will end and I will walk again soon *out there* in the crisp October. But her voice is far away. I have never been so completely inside a room, dull in the delirium of my body. I am stretched skin, I am mucus, I am tongue receiving breath. I squat back into the next contraction, letting my jaw moan loose. A deep rumble quakes in the back of my throat, a circular sound I've practiced like *om*. When my voice creeps up to the roof of my mouth and whistles out my nose like a high whine, my doula, Joan, hums a peach-pit growl to draw me down again, the way a choir conductor gives a middle C. There's my pitch. I echo it back. Throat sound, gravity sound, baby-out sound. Low low low, down down down. I barely push into my bottom, a diamond-field of pressure where my pelvis squeezes my baby's cranium. Not pretty sounds, my grunts and groans. For the first time I don't care.

Lloyd sits by my head, saying words like *amazing* or saying nothing. He is my rock here, and rocks don't need to talk. There's his hand on my back, there's his blue-veined foot in a brown flip-flop. A hand brings a straw to my lips, and I sip spurts. Icy peanut butter and banana. When the next contraction crests, heat ripples down below. Call it my vagina or my anus—I can't differentiate anymore—they're one bulging cliff face. I roll back into a squat.

"Ring of fire, I feel the ring of fire," I say.

"Good. That's so goood," my midwife coos. "Listen to your body."

I barely push again when suddenly I feel a gush, like a soggy paper lunch bag whose bottom drops out. Sploosh. Then a cry surprises me, loud and opening wider. A new voice. Could it be? I turn my head to look behind me, and between powder blue gloves, my midwife holds my baby, wiping my blood off his head with a towel. I gasp, my relief as big as my surprise.

34

An hour later, my midwife, Lydia, draws a picture for me.

"Here's your vagina. Your tear goes in two directions. Down the middle and up to the side." It looks like a wobbly L turned upside down. I lay naked in my bed while my legs butterfly open onto a nest of pillows. Lumped on my chest is my baby, my second son. I glance at the one-armed stick figure on a paper towel that depicts my genitals, but nothing my midwife is saying matters much right now. In blue skies and clouds, her voice flits flight attendant calm, *Seat backs and tray tables in their full upright and locked positions.*

"The tear is second degree, meaning not just skin but muscle has torn too," Lydia is telling me. "A tear going in two directions can take longer to heal."

I nod along, giddy on what I have done, my herculean feat of uterus and vagina. *Of course I have torn!* I think, busting with awe. *My baby is ten and a half pounds! His head is 99th percentile!*

"Do you want me to tell you what I'm doing, or do you want to be distracted?" Lydia asks, needle and suture in her gloved hands at the foot of my bed.

"Tell me what you're doing." Under no circumstances do I want something to hurt without understanding why.

When I see the long needle with the lidocaine and visualize where she is about to insert it, I remind myself, *You are a badass woman who just pushed a ten-and-a-half-pound human out of your vagina; you are not a six-year-old girl getting your ears pierced at the mall.*

The needle pierces my labia, and I squeeze Lloyd's hand. I breathe in. I am alive.

The pregnancy had been hard.

"I wanted to be further in my healing before another baby," I told my therapist, Kristen. My fibers tightened in me, saying, *I'm not ready to do this again. I'm not ready. I'm not ready.* Guider was eighteen months old when I found out I had a surprise baby coming, and I still felt as if I were sitting in a waiting room of motherhood, hoping that someone would call my name, and I would arise and say, *Yes, that's me. Here I am.*

I wanted a second child, but I wanted to be a different mother by the time that child arrived. Not the mother who felt like a monster when she held her baby down limb by limb to strap him in his car seat while he wailed and kicked, wondering if I was violating his sense of bodily autonomy. I knew mothers sometimes needed to move forward with confident purpose in these moments of bodily care, but a rush of simultaneous anger and shame washed over me whenever I needed to use any force in order to protect him in a way that he couldn't understand.

In a dream I held him to my chest, and I looked at his delicate face. Then suddenly I noticed something was wrong: a long wall of ice towered between us. My arms were stiffly inserted in two holes cut in the ice, and through those chilled sleeves, I cradled my baby. He slept cuddled against me, trusting that he was snuggled against his mother's breast, not knowing he was actually nestled into ice.

Like the bewildered blur of descending into abuse, there was no one moment to which I could point and say, *Aha, now I know that I am not fine.* I'd asked my doctor to prescribe me medication for anxiety, but I let the prescription expire. I called the office and asked her to prescribe me medication for anxiety again, just in case. I seemed to stay just within the window of tolerance, always keeping the metric close that medication was necessary *if my anxiety interfered with my ability to complete daily activities*, as my doctor defined it. I could blend organic sweet potatoes into a puree for popsicles to soothe my toddler's teething, and these details of my functioning I tallied in my mind.

Meanwhile, I felt disturbed by the growth of my baby within me as his fingers and toes grew. I was being touched from the inside, tickled in places I couldn't name by body parts I couldn't see. What was that sensation—a fingering of my cervix, a fiddling of my placenta, an elbow against my bladder? I wanted to know where I was being touched and by what.

One day in my second pregnancy when Lloyd came home from work, I knew I needed to get out of the house alone, but all I had the energy to do was to drive to a playground parking lot and cry. When I came home, I told Lloyd, "If I can't shake this feeling in two weeks, promise me that you'll tell me I need to get on medication." I managed to shake it once again.

Now, Lloyd stands at the side of the bed and helps me pull myself up to standing. Each slight turn and shift in my weight sends ribbons of heat through my genitals. Once I get to my feet, my whole body feels gaping and unfinished, like skyrise scaffolding, as if all my organs might slip out and fall two hundred feet. I hunch over and curve my spine so that my innards pool in my center rather than drip out of me. I waddle and shuffle, keeping my thighs still and slowly swinging out from my knee. *Left foot. Right foot. Left foot. Right.* A wind-up tight-rope walker marching at a geriatric speed.

"It feels like my baby's head is still between my butt cheeks. Why does it feel like my baby's head is still between my butt cheeks?" I ask, straining to get the words out.

"The swelling," Lydia says.

Once I make it to the bathroom, I lean my weight over the fake white marble and heave, finally able to take in air. My body's elevation has changed. My head is somewhere in the clouds, my torso stretched like taffy, and somewhere far below, in a molten place, is my vagina.

I gradually lower into a squat, just enough to aim for the toilet bowl. By each degree I lower myself, the heat of my vagina pulses. The lower I get, the more it feels as if I am sitting on barbed wire, each coil of the sutures pulling against flesh. The urine stings when it trickles out, and my body flinches to stop the flow. I breathe out and relax my muscles to let it out again, but each rivulet burns. *Loose jaw. Soft. Open.* The same words that got the baby out.

No toilet paper, Lydia had said. Just rinse with the peri bottle. The water is warm, heavenly warm, and it rinses the stinging away.

Lloyd wipes up the blood that trickled down onto the white tile of our bathroom floor. He balls up the towel and carries it to the laundry room.

There is my newborn baby, and there is my newborn vagina. I'm supposed to stay horizontal in bed to alleviate the swelling and to encourage healing. There's an electric charge to my vagina that still throbs with all the good it's done. I want to pat it and say, *Good girl. You are the way love enters the universe.*

It's time for my first bath, and I grip Lloyd's arms like a walker to enter the tub. He braces his feet and begins to lower into a squat with me. My vulva is a band of barbed wire. "No, no, wait, slower," I say, crimping my knees in tiny increments.

A Second-Degree Wound

The room radiates out from my vulva into ripples across the terracotta wall tiles. I remember to breathe. *It's okay. Women do this every day. It will be okay.*
I lean back in the tub, and I move my right hand down to wash my vulva. My whole pelvic hinge is still inflated with pain. I map the border, determining what level of pressure is comfortable. I rub an algae-like layer of lochia delicately with my fingers as I break up the hair clumped with dried blood.
Something strange begins to happen. As my fingers move across my vulva, I can't tell what I'm touching. Communication between my fingers and my brain short-circuits, as if I'm touching a different person's body. I don't recognize an inch of it. I touch flesh that is foreign to me; I am far away. There is no picture in my head of what I am touching. *Is this suture or skin? Is this ridge from the birth tear or was this there before?* I can make no comparison of the flesh before the birth and after, unable to acknowledge the changes in an organized, logical way.
My right hand had memorized this vulva land over years of tending. It knew the exact curve where my vagina blended into my perineum. It would follow the trail like a well-worn path. But now, it is as if my hand is the hand of a blind woman meeting a new face. Except I am supposed to know this face. This is supposed to be my own face. I tamp down panic. What I see above the water are unmistakably my own legs, but below the water, what only my fingers can see, is an unclear shape that destroys my sense of what is me.
I only know it's my body because it hurts when I touch it.

A week after birth, my midwife stops by to check on me and the baby. In my bed, I oyster my legs open, and without laying a hand on me, she peers in with a flashlight. I am surprised to hear her voice chirp, "It all looks good. Healing nicely." Her eyes are smiling.

"Hmm," I hear myself hum up into soprano. "Great."

"There's still a good bit of swelling, so stay horizontal as much as possible," she adds. In spite of my shucked-open rawness, I begin to digest that this is what *looking good* feels like. This is functional pain, the pain of creation and healing, *pain with a purpose*, as people say about birth.

After Lydia leaves, I open my baby's memory book to see what she wrote:

I am honored to have been there at your moment of victory.

Maybe I should feel higher than I do—more mountaintop and less salt of the earth. Less serrated and creature from the vagina lagoon. I got exactly what I wanted. A ten-hour labor, a quick dilation, a short pushing phase, a pink-plump second son. "That's the smoothest VBAC I've ever seen," Joan said. "A textbook birth," Lydia declared. So I nudge myself toward the stance of the warrior in the victory, making the connection that for any warrior, there is blood, open flesh, raging capillaries.

On Etsy I'd seen cards that said, *Congrats on your new baby. Condolences to your vagina.* And *your vag is going to look like a bloodhound in a wind tunnel. But congratulations!* I am glad we can give each other cottage-made cards about vaginas and the painfully awkward changes of the body after birth. But the messages now feel as weak as skim milk. What has actually happened to my body is something of a different substance. It is as if I have moved to the rainforest, a wildly divergent landscape from the deciduous forest of Mississippi.

But no one will acknowledge that I have moved to the rain-forest, a place where I have never been before. I live here now. My baby's bassinet lies just beyond the tangle of vines that clasps between my legs.

squirrel

By the time I was sixteen, by the time I met J, my favorite word was *wanderlust*. My mom, a flight attendant,
would call me from the jump seat: *Okay, sweetie, I'll talk
to you later. We're about to close the doors. I've got two more
legs to go.* Cincinnati blurred to Phoenix; Phoenix blurred
to San Diego. She'd spent her early years traveling Europe
and North Africa in a white Volkswagen Bug with Nana,
sometimes sleeping in the back seat of the car with their
dog Missy, using beach showers to bathe and launder their
clothing. Mom's second home was the sky. When I got my
driver's license and my first purple flip phone, I recorded my
voicemail greeting to say, *Bonjour, mes amis. Your nomadic
friend can't come to the phone right now.*

But there was something else I yearned for that I hadn't
yet known: roots. Roots deep as oak trees, roots deep as
hundred-foot pines.

When I graduated from high school, Mom and Nana
packed up our Jackson house and got rid of whatever they
couldn't sell for a dollar at the yard sale. They headed west to
California, where my mom's pilot boyfriend lived. I stayed.

The House of Song sagged atop Jackson's highest hills in one of the oldest neighborhoods in the city. A couple streets over, Greek Revival and Queen Anne mansions towered, but they were fading glories, Southern belles mottled by time and lifetimes of loss. The sidewalks looked like bridges of cards shuffled by massive oak roots and Yazoo clay.

J and I had been together for one year, long enough for me to visit his memaw's house in the country where she served us homemade biscuits; long enough for J to take me to his father's grave; long enough for us to have arguments about me sitting through his mob movies while he tapped his foot and sighed through my romances and dramas; long enough for him to scare me with forevers like *I want you to have my babies*; long enough for me to send him emails with worries like: *I don't know if I could ever spend my life with someone who doesn't like poetry or try new food or look at the stars*; long enough for him to reply saying: *I give up. All I can say is that I love you. I'm sorry if I'm not what you're looking for. Go back to your family if you need to. I just want you to be happy. You deserve to be happy.*

I moved into an all girls' dorm one mile from the House of Song, but on the weekend, I woke up secretly in the little white house. J took his glasses off to sleep, and so did I, our heads on pillows next to each other, Red's velvet at our legs. I'd never seen dawn at the House of Song before. I woke up close to his eyelashes, kissed his forehead, and skipped down the front steps to the Mississippi sky that awaited me.

In late August, two weeks after college began, Hurricane Katrina ravaged the Gulf Coast. It knocked out the power and water all the way to the center of the state in Jackson.

After driving through the post-Katrina neighborhood where power lines snaked the asphalt, my roommate Mary and I hunkered down at a hurricane party. We entered a blur of weed smoke, neon lights, music from a speaker generated by the power of a red Ford pickup, and the gloss of *Playboy* issues, which we flipped through with anthropological fascination.

Mary and I had met in high school in the Mississippi Girlchoir, and we quickly became close since moving in together. Mary's energy was bright and grounded, with mischief radiating from her dimpled, cherubic cheeks. Before long, we went almost everywhere together on campus, except she turned right at the sidewalk fork into the science buildings (psychology) and I turned left toward the humanities (English and French). We were two curly-black-haired, Converse-wearing, subculture twins. When we walked through the dorm halls, we made escalating, orgasmic moans before busting out in laughter.

After the hurricane party, we slept at her parents' house. My phone stopped working in the mess of power lines and rainfall, and I felt free. On the edge of the raging hurricane, I felt free.

Two days later, I went to J.

"You couldn't have called me? You couldn't have just let me know you were okay? Cathy, I was worried sick about you. You can't just disappear from someone you love."

Some red flags are delivered like a bouquet of red roses, a sign of being loved and mattering to someone so deeply. J needed me. My *boyfriend* needed me. I liked the idea of it. But sometimes if I didn't answer my phone, he would panic and call me ten more times. Whenever I wasn't staying over at his house, he began calling incessantly for reassurance that

I loved him, that I wasn't doing anything stupid, that I was where I said I was—not out drinking with college boys.

I apologized for disappearing and promised I'd be more responsive in the future. Then his eyes lit up as he told me about two baby squirrels he'd found near his front steps after the storm. Their nest had been blown out of a tree, so J brought them inside and wrapped them in a warm towel. One hadn't made it through the night, but the other was snuggled in a washcloth in a shoebox. He opened the lid to show me. The gray baby curled in the palm of my hand. J had already bought kitten formula and fed it with a syringe, a tenderness that warmed me through. I squeezed his palm three times. *I. love. you.*

Loud music rolled. Prince, Bowie, and Queen. The photography studio was a small, windowless room with a roll of white vinyl hanging from the ceiling. A new friend had told me about a photographer named Josh who was making a portrait series of nude bodies painted in a spectrum of colors, A to Z. She'd just modeled for him, skin electric blue. Right away I asked, "Is he looking for other models?"

I chose seafoam green. I undressed and spread my body across a foldout table. My friend used eye shadow to make my face a cosmic-oceanic purple and turquoise, and Josh painted all of my skin with seafoam circles and triangles. We stayed in the studio until 3 a.m. At the end, I poured a bucket of paint down my front and ran my nails across my chest like claw marks, fierce and free.

I hadn't told J my plans. I wasn't expecting him to be pleased, but when I shared about my night, he seethed.

"I can't believe you fucking did that," he said. "The thought of that little leprechaun man seeing you naked and touching your body disgusts me."

"He only touched me with a paintbrush. And it was professional," I clarified.

Our conversation began to feel like girlhood in my dad's house. After Mom became a flight attendant, Dad relentlessly missed her. Our hours home alone remain in my memory as an endless stream of Dad's voice, a radio I couldn't turn down or escape: *She should be here. This is ridiculous—we need her.* And the channel that stung the most: *She doesn't care about us; if she cared, she would be here.* In my mind, his voice went prime time for hours, and even if I retreated to my room for homework, a few minutes later, he would appear in my doorway with subheadings and counterpoints.

I learned that the emotional needs of men can be heavy and ankle-rubbing clasps. I learned that a woman's freedom and independent joy can be scattershot to a man's stability. Perhaps most damaging, I learned that there was no use in trying to challenge a crazed man's voice, no matter how angry I was. Nodding my head and agreeing could end it all faster.

Dad didn't know it, but Mom and I could be free anyway, secretly, and this freedom was our private oxygen, outside the jurisdiction of any man's control. Mom had a small book with a hot-pink patent-leather cover called *The Bad Girl's Guide to the Open Road*. We sometimes locked eyes with a twinkle and said simultaneously, *It's time to hit the road*, and within minutes, her bare foot was propped on the driver's seat with her knee leaning out the open window.

My relationship with J was still something I kept hidden from my father like a snow globe I could shake in the back of my closet. In this way, love was mine, all mine, this shimmering world where he had no say. But as J unspooled into displeasure about the nude photos, I was beginning to realize that just as I'd seen between my dad and my mom, whatever enlivened me and felt like sky would become a threat once J saw it.

My philosophy professor, Dr. Hopkins, required all the freshmen to come to his office for a casual check-in. Our conversation gravitated toward my boyfriend and how he didn't want me to go to parties or drink alcohol and how he made fun of my new friends, calling them bad influences. Dr. Hopkins looked at me with the same level focus on his face as when he taught us about *red herrings, straw men,* and *ad hominem.*

"How would you feel if you broke up tomorrow?" Dr. Hopkins asked.

"Relieved," I said. The word lifted off my shoulders with wings. But it felt traitorous once off my tongue. J was the shape of home, of leaving the light on, especially now that Mom and Nana were almost two thousand miles away.

But my mind tracked back to how even in our first months of dating, I'd written in my journal about *an aching feeling that I'm losing myself.* Nana sat with me on the back porch and shared, *Catherine, you lost your spark since you met him. You don't dream anymore. You don't write anymore. I like J, but he's lifeless. He's not inspiring.* I'd swallowed those concerns, believing that my spark was more bonfire than candlewick, not a fire that a man could fit in his hands, not a fire he could extinguish.

Except he was starting to ask for more of my oxygen, and he was getting scared and angry when I didn't give it to him. *Relieved.*

I knew what I needed to do.

The next day, I walked into his bedroom, and he sat at his computer playing *World of Warcraft*, pausing his finger strokes to smoke a Winston. "Why are you doing this to us?" J said, with an accusatory disdain. He said it again, this time unraveled into a plea: "Why are you doing this to us, Cathy?"

I stayed firm in my plan, even though it felled me to break his heart, even though my heart was breaking too. I could feel it on his skin: His fear of abandonment, the way he'd been hurt by his brother's alcoholism, and the fear of mortality that took root in him after his father's death. I saw his pain in its complexity, and I wanted him to know that I loved him anyway, that he was deserving of love. But I saw no way forward for us, no bridge between my freedom and his fears, my sky and his wall.

"You'll abandon everyone who loves you, just like your mom," he sputtered. "Just go." When I shut the front door to the House of Song, I didn't feel relieved. I felt cruel, my heart blown to the ground. I felt his cruelty too. I'd shared my private pain that I missed my mom when she flew, that even as a mature teen, I still needed her and didn't deserve the brunt of Dad's loneliness.

The next night Mary and I were invited to smoke pot in a stranger's dorm room. We sat in a circle on the floor with neon lights illuminating the faces around me. I'd never used a water bong, and the gurgling unsettled me, along with the smell of funk. Blind Melon came on the college boy's stereo, and I opened into tears. We sang that one together, J and I, and when we sang, I felt like I could survive anything, roots to outbalance a hurricane. Suddenly, I felt my gut lurch in this room with the boys whose unfamiliar teeth glinted in the neon lights. I could hear J's voice in my head. *For this, Cathy? This is why you gave us up—for some puny losers who probably can't even remember your name? What we had was so special; just wait, you'll see.* I wanted to get out of there.

Squirrels build their nests in the tree branches twenty feet or higher. Made of clumps of leaves, twigs, bark, and moss, the nests often rest in the fork of a branch or against a cavity in the wood. Squirrels work with the natural architecture to create their own protective structure.

J and I got back together the next day at the House of Song. A little white house with paint curling by the door, two dogs on the couch. Music and artists and my perfect feet. Singing in bed, singing in hallways, singing at stoplights.

But after I left and came back, something was different. I understood that he wanted me in a way that I could not give without taking my own air. That, equally, our love was a nest, without which I felt groundless. I wanted to burrow into that cavity and feel safe and warm, to lean my body into the curve of a bigger body where the branches intersected.

Maybe, I thought, there is no home without a corresponding desire to leave home. Maybe this is what love feels like.

My favorite high school English teacher, Mrs. Graham, had given me a novel called *Fugitive Pieces* as a graduation gift. Anne Michaels writes: "I couldn't turn my anguish from the precise moment of death. I was focused on that historical split second: the tableau of the haunting trinity—perpetrator, victim, witness. But at what moment does wood become stone, peat become coal, limestone become marble? The gradual instant."

I cannot remember the moment when I started lying to him. I can't make a clean line through the half-truths and the unmentionables, the omissions and the pretending, to put a finger on the precise moment when I was no longer more in love than I wanted my freedom. I began lying to J, but it didn't feel wrong. There was a truth I was telling: that my freedom is an inside job. The women in my family share this freedom only with each other; it's not the men's business. There are demands from men that we pretend to oblige, but in secret we tend to our own agency. I'd never seen a man fully accept the wide freedom of a woman he loved, and as far as I knew, it wasn't possible.

So I went to the Heaven and Hell party at the Lambda Chi house. I dressed as Heaven, all lacy white with a halo. Or maybe I dressed as Hell, red dress, red lips, and black hair. I can't remember; those details crouch in the shadow of secrets. I got crushes on boys who played guitar way worse than J, chords clumsy and trite, and though I never kissed them, I sprawled across their top bunks with Mary, and our eyes edged with desire. I drank beer, I drank the red punch from the cooler, I drank gin and tonic, I drank tequila shots, I drank rum and coke. I lived the way I wanted to live, and I kept that from J. I kept it for myself, my own private world. I leaped up the steps to the House of Song, returning with the flushness of someone well oxygenated.

He said to me, "Cathy, don't ever become one of those middle-aged women scowling at the grocery store." He'd seen it in his own mother as she checked the labels on boxes, a general displeasure for the ingredients of life as a woman. I promised him I wouldn't. Not ever. He still brought up the nude mermaid photos anytime we had an argument. "Fucking disgusting. I thought you were better than that." Even when I disappointed him, I still kept my home in the sky.

Eventually it was time to let our Katrina squirrel go. We opened the front door and placed him on the concrete stoop. He just sat there for one minute and then two, looking at us with his bushy tail in the air. We closed the door. He scratched on the door. Oh god, he scratched on the door. But we couldn't keep him. He was pooping all over the couch and the carpet, and he needed to be in the wild.

It was the mood of that time that we would, together, save a wild, dying thing and nurse it until it no longer knew how to leave us. We watched out the front window until our squirrel leaped off the stoop, across the grass, and into an oak tree.

PRIVATE PARTS

I stand in the bathroom and hold a red compact mirror in my palm. The case is jeweled and glazed in red glitter, which makes me think *There's no place like home* every time I click it shut. Short red ribbons hold the magnetized sides together, and I open the mirror like a drawbridge, bend my knees until my legs spread shakily, and look.

My god. My vagina is a trench coat now. My vagina is like a big fish's mouth left open, hooked and bleeding. The lines come to me fully formed, poetry a reflex.

My mind jumps to what my friend Suzanne told me two years earlier in my first pregnancy.

"Whatever you do, don't look down there after birth," she said. "Trust me. I made the mistake of looking and . . . I can't unsee it. I'll never see it the same way again."

"What did it look like?"

"Wrecked. Unrecognizable. Huge. Wide open. But it got better."

I didn't end up needing that advice two years ago because my first baby was not born through my vagina. But now, between my black curls and the merlot-dried blood, I wish I had one more hand to shine my cellphone light up there for a clearer look. From what I can see, everything is wider. Canyoned. The lips are long dough that's been rolled out. I reposition one side lightly with my thumb and forefinger, and it retains the shape. Before, my lips met at the center and closed into one clean line that held tight to my body, girlish. Today they are parted wide like elevator doors stuck open, and I peer into the raw sheen.

The strange new configuration reminds me of a paper-doll puzzle my toddler has where he can affix the head of a fireman on the chest of a construction worker and the legs of a policeman. It's as if a horizontal strip of my body has been taken out and traded for someone else's. I can't help but feel that the vulva that was mine for thirty-one years is still mixed up in the box with the other pieces somewhere. I wonder if my lips will close. I wonder if this is what people mean when they say *loose*. I don't want to unsee it.

My in-laws order takeout, and I shuffle to the dining room for the first time. The table is set with plastic containers dewed with steam on the lids. Lloyd stacks two thin throw pillows on my wooden chair, but when I lower myself, the contact with the seat sends a shudder through my body. I am sitting on electricity. Heat bolts my tear.

I look around the table to see if anyone can tell that I am melting, but my family looks normal. Panorama of toddler chatter, grandmother smiles, and plastic spoons of potato soup. Baby Rowan is asleep in the swing. I used to think love might feel like this, a family contained around the table with a hot dinner and a baby rocked asleep. I wasn't wrong—love does look and feel like this. But it also feels like I am leaking pain-heat from carefully folded insides, and I am the only one who is leaking. Only stranger than the liquid ruby of my body is the reality that motherhood is an encounter of isolation. I can be in a room full of loved ones and feel entirely separate, smuggled inside the singular experience of The Mother, attuned to my baby's and toddler's every sound. I am the one alone with my past too.

A memory from my first postpartum: There was a night when I rocked Guider to sleep, the room dark, save for the hall light. I began singing the first words that came to me, lines from a Pink Floyd tune–turned–lullaby. J and I used to sing it while he slowly strummed with his fingertips, our eyes nodding each other forward into harmony, into unison. Summer days when clocks melted, golden sunsets gently died, and his palm rubbed my shoulder.

Guider and I, we were welded by our sweat, his head finally heavy and sinking into my chest. I didn't want J anywhere near my baby, but on that night, I saw that the songs I knew best were the music we'd made together, where my voice had lain next to his in the harmonies. I'd avoided the songs for years, but now I found that my voice needed these words, this melody.

"Your voice is so beautiful," my mother-in-law gushed from the doorway. "He is so lucky to have a mother like you." A density compacted suddenly in my belly, a striation of memory.

She didn't know that in my head I was wondering: *Was it J's song? Was it ours?* There was air we passed back and forth over these lyrics. Something like comfort, something like safety, something like love. But also a dark surge of silence, something like my center drowning.

On day eight of Rowan's life, he begins to cough. If he were a newborn cat, his eyes might not even be open yet, so I won't try the echinacea, calendula, and lemon-balm tincture, not on this barely born son. We've taken it as far as a cool mist humidifier can take us. Lloyd drives us to the pediatrician's office.

"I hate to have to tell you this, but I think he needs to be admitted," his doctor says, diagnosing RSV. "It's likely to get worse before it gets better." I think of the two giant bottles of hand sanitizer at our front door and how he's hardly left my chest. I think about the dangerous things that catch us when we think we're safe. We drive home to pack a bag for the hospital.

I am aware that this will challenge my plan to stay horizontal in bed as much as possible. My vagina feels heavily starched as I think about the foldout couch and the pacing back and forth across the tiles when Rowan cries. Another part of me wonders how I could be thinking of my vagina in a time like this.

Born at home. Home birth. Born at home, we say over and over when we check in. We live in a part of the country where only a few doctors will deliver a baby vaginally after a C-section, so I try to compensate by showing the doctors and nurses how well I can retain words like *apnea* and *bronchiolitis* and repeat them back in cogent questions. I feel like someone trying to walk a line on the shoulder of the highway without staggering. *Yes, I am sane. Yes, I am responsible. Yes, I can tell you how many wet diapers he's had today.*

The nurse comes in to get vitals and fluids started. She tapes a pulse oximeter to Rowan's foot and an IV catheter to the back of his hand. I always hate this part: the restraint of baby bodies that don't yet understand that it's for their own good, the grip, the needling, the hold. The nurse wraps his hand in a swaddle of gauze until he has a huge puppy paw that he can barely lift. Next, cannulas spill from his nostrils, and clear tubes are taped to his cheeks with white squares. He wriggle-wrestles against the cords. The tiniest blood pressure cuff in the basket hovers in to squeeze his bicep that's fuzzed with black hairs.

"This is going to hug your arm," the nurse says sweetly as her voice escalates into baby talk. They'd said it to Guider, too, when he was hospitalized with pneumonia in the spring. As Rowan's mouth becomes swollen with cries, I feel the manifesto rising in my head, the one about the sneaky ways we imprint on children that unwanted touch is affection. Suddenly it feels as if someone has wrapped a hot washcloth around my neck, the heat rising to lick my cheeks. I try not to imagine what my child is learning about what a big body can do to a small body when it thinks it has the right. How they'll call what hurts you a hug.

You're so brave. You did so good, they rave when it's over. Only if the child doesn't scream or try to bite them.

Lloyd sets up a pallet for me on the foldout couch, with two giant yoga bolsters that help me take the pressure off my vagina. Beyond the metal grate of the crib, I watch Rowan's oxygen numbers crawl up and down the upper eighties, hoping for the oxygen to tip him over ninety. I play a French lullaby from my phone's speaker: *Dodo, l'enfant do. Sleep, baby sleep.*

Even when I sleep, it's as if the eye of my vagina stays open.

Before I became a mother, it had hardly occurred to me that I would have a son. The force of my future daughters felt vibrant in me, growing in my womb before the sperm had a chance to take root. After I knew there was a baby, I sensed the future rippling under my skin. *My daughter.*

How would I mother a son? While I had close relationships with the women in my family, my bond with my male kin centered around adequate tire pressure, an armory of police-grade Mace, and heavy metal flashlights that could be used either to survive a natural disaster or to club a man. I had close friendships with men and had married a sensitive man, but the model for sharing blood intimacy with a male was not within me.

After my first baby was born, I changed his diaper and softly wiped his penis, squishy and vulnerable, like a baby mole with its eyes closed. With my finger, I lifted his penis so I could wipe the scrotal ridges underneath, smushed small as thumbprints; and his testicles shifted like two rolling marbles in a pouch. I did this eight to ten times a day.

One day as I stood at the changing table over him, his wide eyes staring up at me, it occurred to me that if I were a person who wanted to put my mouth on a baby's penis, I would have that terrible power here, all alone in this house. And no one would know. The thought, although light and passing like a cloud, disturbed me, and I immediately shook it off. I knew I would never do that to any child, but did normal people have these images flash through their head? I'd gone through trainings as a private school teacher, courses with names like Safeguarding God's Children and Darkness to Light. I'd already thought about the ways I could take action to keep my kid safe against sexual abuse. I had a toolkit ready to deploy.

But being alone in the house with my baby hour after hour, day after day, felt insidious. The isolation stirred up shame, times of hiding and secrets and lies. I could feel myself returning to a closed-doors place with private moments no eyes but my own had seen.

At the changing table, I watched my son's penis inflate suddenly and spray pee around the room like a dancing cobra head. I quickly grabbed a cloth and tossed it on top of his spray. These are the kinds of moments other mothers laugh about, I thought. There are even products called Peepee Teepees that look like chipmunk-sized cotton party hats, with the sole function of preventing your penised infant from peeing on you. But my baby's upright penis sent my thoughts somewhere else.

It's easy to tolerate the idea of my baby's penis. A baby penis is innocent, nonthreatening, a kind and silent traveler. But a baby penis will grow into a six-year-old penis, will grow into a twelve-year-old penis, will grow into a sixteen-year-old penis and a twenty-five-year-old penis. A baby's penis will hopefully one day become the penis of a middle-aged man and then an elderly man, or who knows, maybe a woman. I'd love her just as much. These are the hopes we have for our children: that their whole bodies will be safely traveled into the fullest measure of the future.

Still, I couldn't keep myself from wondering: Will my son ever hurt someone the way I was hurt? Will his body ever become a weapon? As much as I wanted to fiercely protect him from outside harm, it felt equally my mission to make sure that he didn't inflict violence.

After four days in the hospital, Rowan is discharged. I push the baby stroller through Target, eyebrows furrowed as I read every ingredient on the back of the all-natural baby wash, phone in hand to Google ingredients I don't recognize. *Glyceryl oleate, tocopherol, phenoxyethanol. Can I trust it, can I really trust it?* On the next aisle over, I spot adorable, fruit-shaped silicone teethers, but when I pull up reviews, I find photos of bitten-off nubs of grape-colored plastic, failures of products marketed as safe. I've already become aware of pockets where mold could hide inside a squishy giraffe, edges that can become sharp on play gyms, and splinters on heirloom wooden rattles. There are materials that haven't yet been identified as dangerous, plastic compounds too pernicious to regulate—*Are we safe? Are we really safe?*

And the answer was: sometimes we're not. In my first pregnancy, unsafe amounts of lead had been discovered in our city water system. Pamphlets arrived warning that pregnant and nursing women, along with children under five, should not consume the water. Unfortunately, I'd already been drinking it for the first half of my pregnancy. No children had become sick from the lead, as far as we knew, but when I rubbed my belly, I feared a swirl of poison.

On the sippy cup aisle, I furrow my brows at the cost of the stainless-steel cups—three times as much as the plastic ones—but I toss two into my cart anyway so that my toddler's water won't marinate in plastic chemicals. Is this what mothers do when we feel we have toxic memories leaking from us, distorted cells that could grow inside our babies like cancer? Is that what we do when we feel dangerous and damaged, threatening and vulnerable at the same time? The violence in my past cooks all around us like microwave rays. Spinning, converting, beeping, steaming.

What I can control is the angle of the tiny nail clippers with the window that helps ensure I won't pinch my baby's finger flesh. I want every one of my decisions to say: *I am your mother, and I will protect you. I am your mother, and I am doing everything in my power to keep you safe.*

My biggest fear when I became a mother was that none of these details mattered because I was failing to do the one thing that was most important: to love my child with the warmth a mother should. My biggest fear was that all I could control would never be enough because a man's penis was forced inside my mouth nine years ago and now I use that mouth to kiss my sons, and why, when I am kissing my baby's head, am I picturing a penis I don't want in my mouth?

Are you loving every minute? a stranger asks me in the checkout line. *Don't blink.*

kudzu

When I was twelve years old, I found the photos of my mother. My eyes landed on a woman in a black leather corset, breasts uncovered and a tan line visible on her upper thigh. On a bed, she sat back on her heels while her chest leaned toward the person behind the camera. Her head was thrown back and her mouth gaped open, not as if she was trying to speak but as if she was making a sound I'd never heard before. She was my mother. But she wasn't my mother. She was a woman I wasn't ever supposed to meet.

I must have been in the house alone because I flipped through the stack of photos slowly, taking in her bared throat, splayed lips, and stroking fingers. In my memory, the photographs blur. Was she in the bathtub in one, as if someone had walked in and surprised her while bubbles covered her waist and her brown nipples gleamed? Was she wearing a high-cut black thong in another, glancing over her shoulder? What remains in my memory is that she looked powerful, but it felt like the kind of power you have when you're inside a cage.

The bright midday light cut through the crepe curtains in our living room, with an intense clarity that tangled with my confusion. The photos were recent. They were taken in the house where we still lived, where we'd lived for only a year. It chilled me that these images were staged behind the same white double doors of the bedroom where my parents fought while I sat on my bed with my teeth chattering, the stained concrete floors in the hall delivering the arguments straight to my door. On the worst night, I'd heard my dad crescendo into words that made me flinch. One word: *slut*. I had sat with my chin tucked between my knees like we'd practiced in tornado drills at school. In my tornado nightmares, the shingles flew off, the wind roared like a train, and I tucked my head while waiting for it to pass, not knowing if the walls would stand when it ended. He wouldn't hit her. He'd never hit us. I was almost certain he would never cross that line, but his words tore through me like a seam ripper.

"Come on, Catherine, let's go." My door had opened. My mother was there, her black carry-on in her hands, her face a blot of mascara, defeat, and heartbreak. She was brazen and she was broken, all at once. My dad's voice was a swirling funnel that followed us, loud and closing in. My heart pelted me, pinging against my breast buds like hail. I stuffed my school uniform into my backpack and grabbed my tooth-brush. Would I even go to school the next day? My dad's voice ricocheted around us like debris, and we ducked our way to the door. In less than two minutes, Mom and I were in her Land Rover, the dashboard lights like fiery flares. My dad, barefoot, stood at the top of the driveway as we started to reverse. "Catherine, you don't have to go!" he called out, wringing his voice into something softer, like a lullaby you might sing to a child as the world is ending. But I was already gone. I furrowed my brows and let my eyes meet his briefly in a way that said, *Sorry*, but then my eyes cut away, and that loss of connection felt like the only justice I could render. As Mom switched from reverse to drive, I looked back at my father. I'd never seen someone so lonely, and his pain ached in me. But how could he think I would stay? The saddest part was that he thought there was still a chance that I might stay. When I looked over at Mom in the darkness, her eyes were empty travelers that watched the road. I swallowed and looked forward too. Mom and I shared a heartbeat. Everything that was hers was mine.

From my dorm room, I walked to my 8 a.m. class, "Love and Sex in the Ancient World." I scrawled spiral-bound notes while my eyelids lazed heavily from the short night of sleep. Even in this half-awake murmur, Sappho's poetry sang to me. Other ancient Greek poets, like Homer, were writing about epic feasts and mythic splendors, but Sappho invoked the significance of ordinary, human love, with heartache and soapy hair.

As I walked out of class and past the classics department offices, I saw a flyer on the bulletin board for a study-abroad trip to Greece. Sixteen days on the mainland and three islands. Early summer. A *yes* flared in me, the kind of yes that awakens you with flint and stone spark. I was summoned. Me in the ancient ruins, standing in the Parthenon amid the vigor of what couldn't be destroyed. Me in the blue and white rousing of Santorini, olive oil slicking my lips. There, too, with newly risen stars above the Minotaur's labyrinth. My dad had told me that with my scholarships, he could pay for me to study abroad every year if I wanted, which was one reason I had stayed in Mississippi. Greece rose in my throat, blooming.

When I told J about it, he rolled his eyes and scoffed. He shook his head as if I was ridiculous and disappointing him. *What a stupid thing to do. What a stupid thing to* want *to do.* All he saw was a college girl on a quest for a boozy Mediterranean cruise. No holy place. No ancient mystery beyond imagining.

Greece became a battlefield between us that he would rampart for months. But I wouldn't retreat. There was nothing wrong with wanting to go to Greece, I laughed right back at him. All I wanted was to visit a true and storied place that exists on this freaking amazing planet. Greece was a reasonable thing to want. He looked at me as if I were a weak poppy bending in a headwind.

Despite my resolve, the way we camped our ranks of foot soldiers on that field for months and fortified our embankments began to change something in me. That my trip to Greece was a problem became a tired fact between us, a land unrooted and booted to mud, a torchless night watch. I stopped trying to defend myself or explain myself by raising my voice or shaking my head. I knew there was no use; we would be back at the same standstill tomorrow. His protests became an annoyance, a chigger thicket, a horsehair rash.

Until one day, he said with a grin, "You know . . . one thing could make this better." His eyes drifted blue, a fluorescent twinkle. "If I could have a video of us together, I could watch it when you're gone. It would help me not miss you so much."

A video.

A sex tape.

I raised my eyebrows and made a sound somewhere between a groan and a sigh. I was pretty certain I never wanted to be president, but I still didn't want a sex tape of me in the world. Paris Hilton's *1 Night in Paris* sex video had been released only two years before, and I'd imagined the horror of my parents seeing me in ruby-throated seduction. Though they'd never instructed me to *wait until marriage*, sometimes while having sex, amid the noises and tastes, I got a flash of my papa watching me from heaven, disappointed in his sweetie straying so far from the little girl who delighted him by singing over her oatmeal. It was as if I started out as someone special and glimmering, but the more I grew, the more I distanced myself from innocence as I became a woman, the more my specialness subtracted toward nothingness.

Before long, J marshaled not around Greece but around the sex tape. I could go to Greece—it was still stupid—but I could go, he said. The problem was actually that I wouldn't make this video, that I wouldn't do this one small thing for him. He'd be fine with Greece if I made the video. I shook my head; day after day, I shook my head.

"Come on, Cathy, you're missing my birthday," he begged. It was true.

I'm not sure of the moment when he backed me across the threshold into the edge of the forest. What I remember is that I wanted desperately to shove something in his mouth to make him stop pushing me across the glut of meadow grass and into the band of wild darkness. I wanted to push him back, even if it was with a part of me that felt more like the nothingness than like my true self.

I was eighteen years old in a black lace thong and a corset that clasped at every spine hold. "Gold Digger" by Kanye played from his computer with revolving slinky tessellations, and I smelled weed sliding under the closed door from his room-mates' rooms. J was holding my camcorder. A grin routed his face. I shimmied toward him where he reclined on the bed in navy boxers. I turned, looked over my shoulder, and shook my ass. I straddled him and leaned forward to swing my breasts near his face, but I didn't let my warmth touch him, not yet. If I hung a smile on my face or not, I don't remember. At my center was my anger and he welcomed himself to it. I felt myself become a woman right there, in this anger. I felt myself churning with my mother, my grandmother, and my aunt, the forces of male control that had looted them and their power that still stood, unbeatable. I spilled my black hair over him, long enough to cover his neck veins, his shadowy mouth, and his blue-shock eyes. He couldn't see my face when I felt his body go quiet.

In Greece, I climbed to the site of the ancient oracle at Delphi, raced across the field where the original games were held in Olympia, and swam in my underwear in the cold Mediterranean Sea by moonlight.

On the trip was Taylor, a musician with a golden pony-tail who fell asleep on my shoulder during miles of bus treks from the raw coast of Mykonos to the misty cliffs of Sparta. Taylor and I had sung together in the college choir, where we both held down the low notes, I an alto to his bass. But on the trip we bonded deeply the way travelers do on a pilgrimage, swapping stories from our childhood, splitting plates of oily pasta, and wandering sacred ruins. On the bus singing *Abbey Road*, on the bus singing Death Cab for Cutie, on the bus singing the Decemberists. Asleep on the bus, sharing chips on the bus, looking out the window shoulder to shoulder. He cut his big toe while racing across the game field in Olympia, and I raised his foot to my lap to swab his big toe with alcohol before bandaging it. If I had kissed that toe, the moment would have felt only slightly more intimate. Taylor also had a serious girlfriend; he bought a lava rock bracelet for her on one of the islands. Still, one night I fell asleep in the king-sized bed next to him and another guy friend, just sleeping.

J had often said, *You don't know how lucky we are to find each other.* Because I was so much younger and dysfunction felt normal in my family's relationships, I believed him. But I journaled furiously and with clarity on the bus now, seeing my life as I wanted it: love after love after love. It wasn't that I wanted to break up with J to be with Taylor; it was that now I knew that I could find love again and feel at home with other people. I'd been putting off the truth, but I couldn't anymore. J wanted to marry me—wanted me all to himself—and I couldn't stomach the way that future looked. My wet warmth, my anger, my lies. His jealous grip, his heavy need, and his fears. I had an appetite for freedom that I'd barely tasted, having gone from my father's house to J's night watch. The feast was in a room I hadn't yet entered but could once more imagine.

Home from Greece, I pulled up to J's dingy white house with a heavy cannonball in my stomach as I switched gears to park. I didn't knock. This was like my own house. I just walked in, and I sat on the faded blue comforter on his bed while he stood. I don't remember if he was lighting a cigarette or if he was fiddling with his computer monitor, but I spoke before I could change my mind.

"We need to talk. I can't be with you anymore," I said, glancing from his face to the window. Nausea rose from my gut to my throat. I'd never broken up with anyone before, and I knew this would really hurt him. He ran his fingers through his frizzy curls, and his jaw tightened. I watched his blue eyes behind his glasses flutter from sadness to rage.

"I knew this would happen," he said, eyes tracking. "That's why I didn't want you to go to *fucking* Greece." He punctuated the end by punching a hole in the wall. I flinched. He said I was a fucking stupid girl who was wasting the only real love I'd ever find to prance after some rich frat boy who just wanted to get in my pants. My eyes fixated on the crushed edge of drywall, a moon shadow of cracks and crumble. I looked at his fist, which was red but not bleeding.

Although he moved slowly, almost lazily, the scene revealed itself faster than I could process it. He threw my car keys behind his TV stand, grabbed me by the arm, and pressed his heaviness on top of me on his bed. He weighed much more than I did, and my ribs were compressed, my breath space shallow. I froze. He lay there on top of me, neither of us saying a word for a few dim breaths. Then he began crying, and it felt as if he was drowning on me. "Don't leave me, don't leave me, Cathy, please don't leave me." I didn't know if his roommates, who were like brothers to me, were home. But I didn't call for help. I didn't even know if I needed to call for help. I didn't know what to call this.

Eventually he stood up, and so did I, but whatever vigor had filled my body in Greece, honey-heavy combs and eaves dripping with berries, had been covered. For three hours he pendulated between shouting at me, something about how he couldn't trust me, a rich girl who didn't know what love felt like, and then crumbling in my arms to cry, "I'm sorry, Cathy, I just love you so much, you're the only thing I have. I can't live without you." Nothing made sense—if I was a horrible person, if I was in danger, if I really did need our relationship, if I would be alone forever.

Then we had sex. I don't remember how it started. I remember only that I cried warm tears that pooled in my ears. I stared at the ceiling with his heaviness holding me down, the hot sprawl of his breath and the silence of my body.

"Why are you crying?" he asked after, with the tenderness of a satiated lover, eyes soft and concerned.

"I just love you." It slipped through my mouth like a roach.

I said whatever I needed to say to find the exit. *I'm sorry.* Promises. Little kiss on the lips. He handed me my keys, and I drove straight to Mary's parents' house.

On Mississippi roads, monsters of green growth tower from the trees, higher than power lines. Kudzu is an invasive species that climbs and coils with dense vines that smother other plants, blocking the sunlight and the root path until they die. Even though it was introduced to the United States as a vine capable of stopping soil erosion, kudzu now has a reputation as a *mile-a-minute invader*. Where it grows, it devours.

J had spent so much time that year wrapping me in words about protecting me from the drinking, the college boys, and the ill intent of the general male population that a profound haze of incoherence blurred me. I had no image of *unsafe* that took this shape: my boyfriend's bedroom, the singing house where I'd passed hundreds of hours, the mattress where I'd rubbed his back when restless legs prickled him in the night. All the images of danger I'd been warned against involved strange men, a hand over my mouth, private tissues ruptured, hard and fast gutting. Not this. No sharp teeth, no claws. Only quiet creeping tendrils smothering me into nothing with hungry green leaves. Flesh I knew to the point of boredom, smells I'd slept against.

I carried police-grade Mace that Dad had supplied, teaching me how to aim low and track up because of a person's instincts to duck. My older brother had taught me how to break out of an armhold; we'd practiced dozens of times one summer, laughing as he gripped my forearm while I jerked down and out in the way that wrenched his thumb joint open. These tactics never welled up in me that day with J, and the violence felt more like humid air all around me than one point of contact to jerk myself out of.

When I arrived at Mary's house and sat on her bed, it was from this shadow of forest-edge twilight that I spoke to her. Undefined shapes halfway up the sky in the pines, muffled sounds that were either mammal tongues or whirring cicadas, dark coils over my shoulder that were either my own braid or a snake. Mary was a psychology major; her eyes moved slowly back and forth while I talked, as if she were reading a textbook that had answers, and in her voice was concern. But I didn't have answers. Not yet. And I couldn't hear hers. I only had the underground root system and the leaves that coated me. The hairs inside my ears still felt slick and wet from my tears, but the sun was setting through Mary's red window tapestry, and it was beautiful against the confusion my story unfurled.

Years later, after I became a mother, my therapist would ask me, "At what point did the relationship become abusive?" Only then would I recognize this day for what it was.

But somewhere below words, I was beginning to sense that my body was an acre J's anger could travel across, and I could disappear somewhere under the canopy, running into the forest toward the wellhead purls. He came to my body as a frantic man, and he left a subdued boy. I almost pitied him. I thought of all the lies I'd told him. I thought of the sex tape, my anger stacked in my vertebrae until I felt more like bone than soft folds of passage. I thought of Greece, where my friends had buried me in the black sand with my hair mermaiding, where Taylor stood a massive phallic stone on my pelvis, and I grinned at the heft of my pubis because the solidness seemed to rise from me, my own. I thought of Fiona Apple using her voice like a blood-wet blade as she sang about being a bad, bad girl who's been careless with a delicate man. Had I pushed him to this place? Had I broken him?

I was my mother's daughter. I was a woman I had not yet seen.

Back at my dad's house that night, I got on my knees and buried my journal from Greece in the plastic bin of Barbies under my bed. I pulled the memory card out of my camera and dumped it under their mass tangle of Velcro dress seams and knotted hair. I clicked the lid closed on top of their smiles and pushed the half-naked bodies into the dark void.

VAGINA GAZING

I lean off the edge of the toilet seat and sniff my underwear, trying to figure out what is leaking from me. I've downscaled from the postpartum mattress pads to panty liners I change every few hours, but I don't have a name for what's coming out of me now. Not the sharp acidity of urine, not the egg-white mucus of ovulation, its slippery stretch on my fingers. This is a clear and watery substance, with only a slight animal musk. It trickles out of me when I stand up from nursing and when I bend to pick up a giraffe rattle from the floor. It must be pee, the way it gushes warm, but it comes independent from any sensation of peeing on myself. It flirts out of the sharp tingle of my urethra (poor girl stretched to oblivion during birth), but the leak is barely an utterance.

I wish the fluid leaking into my underwear were the only mystery. But there's also the question of my butthole. Where is it exactly? In the shower as I swipe my fingers between my cheeks, there's a new rubbery stretch to the skin there, like a balloon that's been filled wide with air and then deflates. When I try to wash myself, it takes me a few tries to find the opening. There are two new pockets of skin that I come to think of as *fool's butthole*. One pocket, I guess, is swollen veins of hemorrhoids. And the other? Some kind of new flap like a ship's sail.

It's an achy vagina day. I try to describe it to Lloyd. "It's as if my vagina has been carrying heavy bags of groceries up flights of stairs." Weighted, full, and painful with yearning. A few minutes later, I find a new way to describe it. "It's like my vulva was injected with warm carbonation." Tingling and prickly. Lloyd nods and widens his eyes in wonder, the curiosity of a lifelong learner, as if I'm telling him about a creature I learned of in the midnight zone of the sea. After all, our wedding guestbook was a tome of old illustrations called *A Cabinet of Natural Curiosities*, and our guests wrote their messages alongside bulbous toad eyes, stinging tentacles, and tubular coral polyps. I belong among them now.

When we first started dating, I remember feeling unashamed as a person with a body, as if the way he looked at me had been wiped clean of the swamp film of the male gaze. "I hope you know you've linked up with someone who would be happy living in a cave with nothing but a blanket," his mother told me with fondness. If you saw Lloyd in our college library, he would look like a straitlaced white boy in a blazer, but if you talked with him, you would know there was heat at his core. His heat wasn't controlled with an on-off switch. More like cave flames licking the wind. Primordial. Essential. Weird. This was the kind of man I knew instinctively didn't care about hair on my legs. He would like my untamed body, my undomesticated mountain. This was the kind of man who would learn my scent and sniff out the trail to me, slinking on hands and knees with his nose leading.

"Are you going to make a man out of him?" a friend jived as we sat on her twin bed with our two best friends, all of us howling with laughter. "I bet he's wild in bed!" she added. I reddened and shook my head. I didn't think about us in those *Cosmo* terms, not the 10 Hot Ways to Turn Him On that you'd see on a magazine cover. It was more like this: with him, for the first time I wasn't caught having a body. Nothing synthetic, nothing invented, only the musk of my underarms on his lips.

When our first son was born, he stayed at my side as I labored on the toilet, where slippery blood and mucus spilled. As I wiped, I couldn't find the end of the slick fluid, like a scarf coming out of a magician's sleeve; I wiped and wiped, and more slickness came, unending. When I felt as if I was finally pushing my baby down, hanging onto the edge of the bathroom door in a squat, I looked behind me on the floor and saw poop, a thin coil, as if from a table-fed terrier. "Oh, I pooped," I said. "Yep, you did," he said. He unrolled a handful of toilet paper, picked it up, and flushed it. On the birthing table he held my right leg back while I pushed, the air smelling like boiled blood and animal exertion. When I was wheeled into surgery, I asked him to narrate the operation for me as a comfort. I expected him to whisper in my ear, "Okay, they're making the first incision now," but instead he veered comedic sportscaster, saying, "Now they're digging out some pieces of corn and flinging ketchup around." He gazed beyond the blue drape, watching all, while the laughter of the whole room tittered off the clamps and scalpels.

Now, as I'm finding new words every day to match the alien sensations of my vagina, I worry that I'm stretching a membrane too thin between us for too long. I'm asking him to absorb the blood, and maybe he's saturated; maybe it's

dripping from the ceiling. I was used to translating myself for
him, the nuances of my body and our touch, origin stories of
my abuses in young womanhood and its legacy of *triggers*.

Months earlier, before Rowan's birth, this: I told him that
when he intercepted me in a hug while I put the dishes away,
I panicked, a feeling of being trapped by J. "I feel like there's
a third person in our marriage," Lloyd said quietly. My eyes
rested on the chipped molding, where dusty blue from
mid-century peeped through the white. Lloyd was beginning his own therapy and *individuation*, separating what was
his from what was mine. He'd been so kind over the years,
holding me and giving me distance and wanting to learn
how to help me feel safe, but I worried I took up too much
space in our relationship. How much is too much pain to ask
your partner to witness? I'm wary of holding it in, but I also
don't want to burden him, every day an armload of charcoal
dropped at his feet.

And now there's my vagina, with its own demands of witnessing. Perhaps there are only so many genital-sensation
analogies I can share before I cross over into the territory of
a wife whose husband *just can't see her in the same way* after
the baby. Or maybe I'm a narcissist, and vagina gazing is just
the hippie sister of navel gazing. But the possibility of all this
isn't strong enough to make me stop. When I lack the language to understand something, I get afraid. I get afraid of
what truth I might be hiding from myself. Like the two years
when I abandoned my journal writing during the darkest
abuse with J.

If I go to this new world of my vagina alone, I am afraid I
will vanish. I don't think Lloyd will be able to find me. Someday I'll hear myself saying, *We just grew apart; we grew in different directions.*

"When I walk, I feel a jiggle inside me," I tell him. "It's like a hard-boiled egg is wobbling at the top of my vagina." His back is to me at the sink, and he squeezes out the sponge.

A postpartum book I read during my second pregnancy recommended taking a picture of your vulva before birth as a reference point for a potential repair or reconstruction. Months ago when I read it, it was spring, and I thought, *No thanks. I don't need a photo. I don't really care what my vulva looks like. Who can even see it under all the hair?*

But I do care. Suddenly I care. Not because I don't think my little cupcake cunt is pretty enough but because my vulva suddenly matters to me and I want to know it. The same way that Lloyd's face matters to me because it is his. I know the spot where his nose meets my face when we kiss, the three long eyebrow hairs that grow wild, the pothole pores from long miles of running under the Mississippi sun. I know the blue flecks of his eyes, light rain streaked on a car window.

Until now I didn't know how little I knew about my vulva. I was satisfied with a pin-the-tail-on-the-donkey, blindfolded understanding of the terrain. I knew what encompassed these three territories: *vulva, labia, vagina.* But what more was there to know? I had a standard-issue vagina. But isn't every girl a little worried that her vagina is the one that barely skated through quality-control inspection, this left lip a little too smushed, that right one a little too long? And we all know the terms: You grow up aware that you could be raped at any moment simply for existing with a vagina, and alongside that, you are aware that a lover might not like the fishy smell. You are aware that a boy is motivated to get in your pants while caring nothing about you as a person.

Conversely, you are aware that what is in your pants might be too gross for anyone to desire. We seesaw on this fear that we could be wanted too much—to the point of violation—or too little—to the point of rejection.

Mothers sometimes say, *My body feels like it's not my own,* and what I'm beginning to wonder now is: when *did* it feel like my own?

I don't have a photo of my vulva before birth. And I wish I did. It's a whole world I'll never see again. I'd like to behold it now and remember, as a mother would.

I lie down on the white shag rug, Lloyd next to me after our kids are asleep. We have three hours max before the baby wakes up again, precious hours of sleep.

"Will you just help me look, please?" I ask. "I can't see what's going on down there when I stand up because it's too dark." I'm not wearing underwear, only the thin layer of my jersey nursing gown. "I can feel what's different when I touch it, but when I look at it, I can't connect what I see to what I feel with my fingers."

He agrees, though unease curves from his mouth. I open and my finger slows as I approach the tender pearl on my vulva that feels like a chewed knot inside my cheek. I point.

"Okay, does this look like it's part of my original vulva structure, or is it new from the repair? Was this there before?"

"I don't know," he says, shaking his head. He leans forward and squints.

"What about this?"

"I don't know."

Over and over again, he doesn't know.

I want to scream. I want to shake him by the shoulders. Well fuck. Who *does* know? *I* don't know. My husband doesn't know. Nine years together and he doesn't have visual recognition? I say none of this, folding back in on myself. I'm not mad at him so much as I'm mad at his shelf-stable body, his organs unaltered while I've morphed into a mutability of hormones and sutures. I'm not mad at him so much as I'm mad at pornified pussies and the images that I pinned in my brain rather than my own vulva's shape.

There are things I want him to understand: that my body feels like the flicker of a neon liquor-store sign, that I feel embedded with shrapnel, that I feel like a colonized land, the grief of never learning my own body, its language, its power, before it was stolen from me. That I was born from the collision of the colonizer's intrusion and the Indigenous forgetting. That my papa grew up in a boarding school set up by the French government in Cambodia to teach the illegitimate children of French soldiers, and he never learned his mother's language, only French. That whenever Papa comes up in conversation with my mom and my nana, one of them asks, *Was it Vietnam or Cambodia?* And I remind them, *Phnom Penh, that's Cambodia.* That if I wanted to know where I was from, then I needed to be the one to memorize the birth certificates or someday our whole history would be lost.

This is what my vulva is asking me to remember too. A language we have forgotten. A body, a home, we never knew.

Lloyd's done. He leaves the room to brush his teeth. I stay on the floor; one heel agitates the shag. A few minutes later he walks down the hall toward our bedroom, and I call him back into the nursery. We stand face-to-face, close enough that we could hug. He is half gone toward sleep, but I am wide awake in this metal-edged density.

"You act like you don't even like looking at my vagina," I whisper so as not to wake our sleeping children. His mouth tugs to the side.

"I don't," he says. "And that's really hard for me to say. I don't know why I don't like looking at it." He has tears in his eyes, but I can't make my arms wrap around him. Damn his honesty. I won't comfort him. I won't get into bed with him and feel him fall into gentle breath beside me. Not right now. I fill the bathtub, remove every layer that can be removed, and sit in there until the water goes cold. I find the flaming pearl with my fingers.

yazoo clay

It's hard to identify my earliest memory, but perhaps it's the impression of being home: rubbing my mother's earlobes while I fell asleep. Soft peach flesh. Honeycomb landing. I squeezed her lobes lightly between my finger pad and thumb, stroking up the cartilage arch. I liked it best when my fingers found her ear cold; I slowly rubbed the chill away. I could also, with a quick series of flicks, fan the lobe from warm to cold in order to have the pleasure of warming it again. My mother says that I first rubbed her ears while I nursed as an infant, and I wouldn't fully wean until I was three years old, a fact that brought her great pride but that embarrassed me whenever she told the story. *Night night*, I called her milk.

I rubbed Nana Jojo's ears as a substitute when I spent the night with her, but she says I was never satisfied with them. I remember how thin and oily Nana's ears felt, like flaps of no substance, narrow anchovies. Still, I remember the courage it took to reach toward her lobes, the strangeness of initiating this specific, intimate touch. I remember missing my mother's body, that no other body could fill that emptiness between my fingers.

I rubbed J's ears the summer I met him, and they were the closest ears to my mother's I could imagine, plump and springy, like my birthday cake coming out of the oven.

It was August, the air so wet and heavy that I could practically drink it. I licked my upper lip as I stood outside, and the sweat-salt felt as if it came from outside me rather than in, atmosphere of a steam room. J picked me up from my dad's house for dinner, but I knew something was off right when I buckled my seatbelt, as certain as the smell of milk gone sour. He didn't say a word when I got in. He took a long drag on his cigarette, his lips strangling the smoke in a sustained release. We'd been fighting more since I came home from Greece, since the night he lay on top of my body and wouldn't let me leave.

"Where are we going?" I asked. When he merged onto the interstate, rather than following the straightaway to the Mexican restaurant, he slowly switched lanes. No answer. I watched his face, a stiff void. Nervousness clotted in my chest, and I realized I was holding my breath. We headed south for ten miles, and although this was the strip of highway I knew best, I didn't know where it would end. He exited at Fortification, the exit for the House of Song. But rather than turning left, he took a right down the steep hill and pulled up to a brick fourplex. It was the new apartment on Peachtree he'd been looking at, the one he wanted to be *our* place. The car stopped completely, and he shifted to park. He sat in silence for a moment.

"Who's Steve?" he asked, his voice low but brittle.

"Steve? Steve's my friend. He works at High Noon," I said, confused. I'd met him when I studied the state's only vegan café for an anthropology project. I sat at the café counter as a participant-observer, recording interactions between regulars and employees.

"I saw your emails, Cathy." J squinted at me as if he already knew the verdict. "If he's just your friend, then why the fuck are you flirting with him?"

Shame rose in me. I guess you could call it flirting, but it felt innocent. Our friendship wasn't different from what I shared with my high school guy friends. Playful, warm, open. Not a threat to my relationship with J. Steve knew I had a boyfriend.

"That's just the way we talk," I explained. "It's nothing more than that."

"This is worse than I thought," he said. "I thought it was just that fucking loser in Greece. Now it's this guy too. I can't trust you."

Although we were not touching, his heart rate felt loud in me.

"It's too bad we won't be able to live here. It's too bad you don't love me," he said, like a threat, as if we were ending. Not just our relationship but our blood flow.

"You were looking at my emails?" I asked.

In a way, part of me had ended. In knowing that he had sliced into the private space of my inbox, an essential piece of me felt cut off, the ventricle that separated me from him. I didn't even know he had the capacity to hack into the college's email system. I stared at the floorboard as unease spread through my body, as if he had power to access every part of me and he wanted me to know it. As if nothing was my own, as if I was a person only in relation to him.

Now, his anger cut in. He grabbed my cellphone from my hand, threw it under his driver's seat, locked the doors, and threatened to make me watch him swallow a whole bottle of pills, the orange plastic in his grip. He started to drive again, and I froze.

Up until then I'd worried about his depression, but his leaning toward death felt more like a cynical worldview than a threat. One time he said, *I'd rather blow my head off than end up old and sick in a hospital with tubes in me, surrounded by strangers. Every man in my family has died of cancer, and the day a doctor tells me I have cancer, I'm going to go home and shoot myself.* I worried about him when he talked like this, but his vigor in railing against our fucked-up health care system or the uneven distribution of wealth loosened my concern. *This isn't Hollywood, Cathy. Soon you'll realize how miserable the world is,* he said. I shook my head, refusing to accept the world as miserable. *Doesn't the fact that I'm so passionate about this turn you on in some way?* he asked, slipping a smile. I scrunched my nose. *What, the fact that you think you're dying? That you're already dead? No, it makes me feel like a necrophiliac.* He laughed. That day our laughter took us all the way home.

But on this day, with the bottle full of pills, there was no laughter. He drove away from the apartment and back toward the interstate. For what seemed like hours, we made laps around the city.

"You're always ruining things. We could just be happy if you stopped doing stupid shit," he spouted as he drove. "Don't you see that all that other stuff doesn't matter, that it's so shallow compared to what we have? Why are you torturing me like this—can't you see how much I love you?"

I calmly tried to talk him down. *Yes, I love you. Yes, I want us to be happy. Yes, I was stupid.* All the while, I kept my eyes on the distance between our car and the bridge railing, our car and opposing highway traffic, our car and the concrete wall. Tears streamed down his face, and I felt his fear of abandonment vibrating off him. I'd seen my dad cry only a couple times, which was more like red eyes than crying. But J felt both liquid and solid, somewhere between boy and man, control and helplessness, vulnerability and violence. His crying felt like a desire for us to be free together, for us to live off the grid of this twenty-first-century nightmare, as if we'd been born hundreds of years too late and were meant for lives bigger than the ones defined for us. It felt as if he were inviting me to build a dream.

"You've hurt me really badly this time, Cathy," he said. "You're going to need to prove yourself to me to regain my trust. It will be difficult, but we can do it because we really love each other, and a love like this doesn't come along every day." I understood that I had caused this pain, and that understanding choked out the other truths: that he had invaded my privacy and that I'd done nothing wrong with Steve. That he needed to regain *my* trust. That I was afraid. That I wanted to get away. But he trapped me in the in-between void, circling his dream until I was exhausted, until the sun gave up and lay down behind the trees.

By the time we got out of the car hours later, I'd agreed to move in with him.

J was more than a boyfriend; he was a biome, the ballad of a whole region. He had shown me the small cabin where his mother was born, the land with a pond where his family had lived for generations, where I got to eat his memaw's homemade biscuits. I'd never set eyes on Algeria's Oran or

Cambodia's Phnom Penh, the cities that grew my grand-parents, but J kissed me in the shade of the cabin where his mother took her first breath, and a shaky part of me steadied.

Though we never talked about it, he was white, and I was white enough to pass, while inside I was something in between that had no name yet. I'd marked *other* a couple times on school forms, but it felt like a betrayal of my family's official story that we were white, so integral that they never explained it. I figured my dad would laugh at me if he knew that I had marked *other*, like a special snowflake. Or maybe he would have been angry. He'd given me his whiteness, and it was mine now, whether I liked it or not. Our whiteness was default; our whiteness was accepted like gravity. And yet, whiteness felt like a half-truth, a white lie of omission, an erasure that voided every other part of my heritage, my mother's side.

Wow, she's so exotic, Mom said her flight attendant friends remarked when she showed them my picture in the galley. I liked being noticed as different, especially in a striking, beautiful way, but *exotic* felt like an aesthetic variant, like wingtip eyeliner. Mom said that somehow the Asian features came out more in me, as if it had skipped a generation; but even then, it felt as if we were analyzing brushstrokes rather than exploring who I was, who we were, something essential about us.

Did I even have a right to call myself anything but white when I couldn't even pronounce my great-grandmother's name? *Thi-Dam Dong.* Mom and Nana laughed every time we tried, devolving into a stereotypical nail salon Vietnam-ese accent to say, *dong ti dong*, like hollow, cheerful bells. I joined them. The distance was so short between her name and our laughter that I couldn't even fit an eighth-note rest between it, couldn't sneak a breath. Nana Jojo also whispered to me in the kitchen, *Shhh, we have some Arabic,* as if she was worried her father would overhear her.

Now I wonder, when your racial identity has a perceptual flexibility and is a sleight of hand, when there's an unspoken narrative of whiteness that's accepted as true by your family while inwardly you feel you're masking difference, when being the only one to see the complexity makes you doubt your own experience, does it make gaslighting feel like home?

Much of the ground in Jackson is made of Yazoo clay. An expansive clay, it expands and swells after rain. When the ground dries, the clay shrivels and shrinks, causing desiccation cracks and suction that can shift tons of concrete. Around here, Yazoo clay is cursed for causing broken house foundations, cracks in plaster walls, and busted car axles from wavy roads and potholes. To remove the clay, the very ground, is not feasible, so builders, engineers, gardeners, and those of us who live here must cope with it. We know heave and shrinkage, downwarping and upswelling.

I knew the fluidity of rearranging my own understanding to make space for an intimate person's perception of reality. I knew the complexity of holding my individual truth separate from the ones I loved. I knew the in-between space of sensing my own feelings while compacting against the swell of another's.

To pay half the rent for the Peachtree apartment, I needed to find a job for the first time. Though I'd never babysat or so much as wiped a toddler's nose, within a couple weeks I'd secured a position as an after-school teacher for three- and four-year-olds. Suddenly I was *Ms. Catherine*, with lesson plans containing words like *gross motor skills* and *manipulatives*. There I was leading circle times and passing out tiny wax cups of goldfish and half bananas still in the peel.

Despite my newness to working with children, I stepped into the role like a mammal who already knew how to mother. The same part of me that was a treasury of my friends' and family's sad stories felt at home amid the breathless wails of children. When I squatted down to look into the eyes of a crying three-year-old, I felt her body hold the entire pain of existence. Under her snot trail and her recess-tangled hair, I witnessed feelings more elemental than a dispute over a knocked-down castle of blocks. This intensity felt like existence itself.

I began receiving invitations to babysit and to spend the whole weekend caring for children during parents' surprise anniversary trips. I learned how to warm up a bottle of breast milk in a bowl of hot water, to change a diaper, to rock a baby and place her gently in the crib. Once you are revealed as a nurturer, those who need nurturing find you.

The kids got picked up by 5:30. By 6:00 I was back at the Peachtree apartment.

One day I walked up while J was strumming on the brick stoop. Red sat at his feet, and she wiggled against me as I sat down. There was no need to announce a song; we knew all the same ones now. He began a Sufjan Stevens tune. I sang along with him, and the neighbor upstairs opened her door to listen.

"You two are so beautiful together," she called down. Her black terrier named Kudzu looked over the railing, tongue wagging.

J's voice was angelic when he took the high notes, white feathers in the breeze. He helped me find the harmony for the chorus, humming me the note, and once I held the note in my own mouth, I hung onto his hum in my ear like latticework. In choir I never wanted to be a soloist, but when we sang together, my voice felt stronger than I ever knew it could be. The music came out of him easy as August rain into the clay earth. My voice grew next to his in the harmonies, crossing over and meeting in the middle. When we sang, I forgot every gap between us that music couldn't fill.

When his voice grew over mine in every place but a song, I held onto the latticework, the echo of my voice. I looked up, squinted, and could see the dream of us reaching toward the sunlight.

BLADDER DIARY

M iddle of winter and the yard's covered in leaf litter, fringed with oaky brown stems and pine straw eyelashes. I throw on my least-stained shirt, stuff my bra with cotton nursing pads, and drive to South Jackson to begin pelvic floor physical therapy. I've lived in Jackson since the onset of puberty, so it's a special day when I need GPS. Today my phone speaks right and left turns from the cupholder as I drive to the edge of my mind's map, where I know I'll meet Veronica, whom my friend Morgan has described as an all-caps QUEEN. When I walk in, I've stepped back twenty years into a community-center gym with machines that have the patina of rubbed metal and sun exposure in a room surrounded by windows. People limp forward on treadmills, lift primary-colored hand weights, and pedal without urgency on stationary bikes.

Veronica, a petite Black woman, retrieves me from the waiting room and walks me down a hallway that becomes darker and uninhabited. We pass through a door that says Pelvic Health. Veronica and I sit down in front of a desktop, and she starts asking me questions. *How many seconds do you usually pee? What's the highest your pain level has been in the past week? Over the past four weeks, how often did you feel sexual desire or interest?*

"I'm noticing you're saying 'I don't know' a lot," Veronica says. "Do you think you have loss of sensation?" Beneath my *I don't know* is a precision of narration I'm seeking, as if I'm having a hard time finding the right word. Above my *I don't know* is the microscopic lens we are now focusing on sensations that have been colossal swaths of texture under my untrained, naked eye. We move through the questions slowly, in a way that feels endless, and although the answers aren't easy to find, I feel myself exhaling, hopeful that answers will come. Not once does she look at me as if I'm an unreliable narrator. Not once does she look at me as if my *I don't know* is weakness.

I undress and she pulls on her gloves. She hands me a plastic model of a pelvis so I can understand where she's touching me, as if I'm holding the round rim of myself and peering in. This brings comfort. She inserts two fingers into my vagina.

"Does this hurt?" she asks. She lightly presses down with her fingers, testing layers of muscle, ligament, and bone. She presses on different points along my inner edges, asking again and again, *Does this hurt?* I respond with *No* or *That feels tender.* Occasionally, *Yes*, it does hurt. Her eyes are kind, receptive. This is different from my encounters with the speculum; finger flesh maps the inside of me, sensate and human. No plastic, no metal. Even as it's happening, relief settles as her hand moves methodically with a cartographer's coordinates. My synapses are connecting, and I can sense the depth and width of my inner corridor, like when my baby found his toes for the first time and realized they were his own body. I'm not left alone with this body and these questions, and I'm not asking Lloyd for answers he doesn't have.

Veronica hands me a big mirror.

"Now bulge lightly like you're having a BM. See that thing coming down on my finger? That's your bladder. You have stage-two bladder prolapse." I am looking at my bladder, and it is sinking into my vagina, an orb dipping like a harvest moon. She gives me a glove and tells me to put my finger inside and bulge again. I watch as I bulge my bladder against my own finger.

Veronica explains that pelvic muscles can become so stressed and weakened in pregnancy and childbirth that they can no longer support your organs. That hard-boiled-egg feeling wobbling at the top of my vagina? It now has a name: *cystocele.*

So often my body exists beyond language, and to learn this word feels like making narrative sense of my flesh. To connect a sensation with a medical reality is sane-making and creates coherence between my own knowing and objective truth. I don't want what I'm feeling to have to be legitimized by professionals in order for me to trust it, but when you've survived gaslighting and abuse, it's hard to have full confidence in your perception. But Veronica is next to me, saying, *You can trust your body's information. I believe you. I see it, too.*

In the doctor's office during the pelvic exams there had always been mystery beyond the peaks of my knees and the folds of the drape, as if that wall of cotton was supposed to barricade us from indecency. But Veronica is close and present, and her words do not feel like chilled metal designed to get in and get out. My stiffness rests into softness; my confidence thickens.

I wish that before I was ever touched by a man sexually, a woman could have walked me through my anatomy with her voice and her hands like this, responsive and matter of fact. Shame has no oxygen here; the dignity of my body fills each corner. I can't help but wonder: what could have been possible if my body had been touched first in a room like this? Or rather, what might have been impossible, unthinkable, because my body was already a solid state in my own hands? I know I can't go back to save her, me at sixteen years old, but I am here in this room today.

Veronica gives me pages of exercises to strengthen my pelvic muscles at home and a few photocopied pages called *a bladder diary*, where I'll track my liquid and food intake, urine and stool output, urgency of elimination, and urine leakage.

"Wouldn't you rather have just had him come out the way Guider did?" Nana asks when I tell her I started pelvic floor PT to regain my strength after pregnancy and birth. She moved back to Jackson when I was pregnant with Rowan, after she left her last boyfriend. She's shown me her own vertical C-section scar since I was a little girl.

"No," I assert, waving my hand. The *no* emerges from my unwavering core. I would choose this intensity all over again rather than the numbness in the year after the cesarean. There is a devotion I am developing to my body now, to its hidden chorus, and I'm beginning to wonder if the victory is not ascension but incarnation, delivery into my own flesh.

Before the pain, my vagina didn't know how to speak, or I didn't know how to listen.

Still, I remember Nana's same voice of concern when she asked me years ago, *Do you see J in your future?* And I hear my voice coyly respond, *The future is tomorrow.* I was seventeen, nimble in my spaghetti straps as I shimmered and evaded her doubts, beaming my smile and confidence that I could manage my future, no threats there.

I know what happened to my body in that future. I know what danger pressed into me, how my lungs squeezed, my breath thinned.

Abuse made me doubt that I was the expert in my experience, possessing the instincts to know if I was lying next to the wolf or the sheep. A part of me still can't trust my perception of reality, fearing it must be the wolf even if my fingers grasp the woolly tufts. My judgments become a fresh absence, an echo in the canyon, and I can't tell if I've just heard the growl of a real wolf on the outside or a scared wolf on the inside, guarding a truth I'm not ready to see.

Even as I feel the hope of reentering my body, I worry about the tricks my mind plays on me, the distortions of memory, the way pain converts into triumph and victims convert into survivors. I worry about repackaging the events that harm us as the events that allow us to be redeemed. Maybe I don't want a moment of victory if it means I will hurt myself along the way.

Each time you leak urine, underline whether you were:

Almost dry   <u>Damp</u>   Wet   Soaked

Activity during leak: <u>Bending over to pick up burp cloth</u>

Was there an urge to urinate? <u>No</u>

As I'm filling out the lines on my bladder diary, I wonder what it would be like if I really heard my bladder's point of view, if

I peeked inside my bladder's private diary. What would it say about the last year, from pregnancy to now? I sit down with a composition book and let my hand lead.

> *It's really cramped in here. I feel like I can't move.*
> *My space is getting smaller and smaller. I'm pressed against*
> *the wall. Someone help me. I'm scared. I don't know*
> *what's happening. I'm leaking. I'm spilling. I can't*
> *control if I stay or go. I don't feel like myself.*

This cry of distress sounds too familiar. I shut the notebook and look out the window at the young magnolia tree, branches bare in the January air. I think about what my friend Lindsey said about emotional abuse: *It feels like someone closes the stage curtains and rearranges the furniture and then opens them again.*

Motherhood has literally rearranged my organs, repositioned my sensations, and altered the construction of my tissues. I find myself looking back to the last place I recognized myself, and I'm reminded of how I looked back after I escaped the abuse, as if I followed a breadcrumb trail asking, *What the hell happened? Where did I go? Where was the last place I saw myself?*

Other times I worry that this obsession with my body's changes is crowding out everything wholesome and happy. Forty-four percent of women have a prolapsed bladder after a vaginal delivery, so common that my doctor didn't even bother mentioning it. Perhaps I am just too sensitive—the line I've internalized since I was a little girl.

But when I begin to worry that I'm too weak and unfit for the world, I remember my strength in birth, the stats that prove my pain tolerance: ten-and-a-half-pound baby, no pain meds, born at home. This helps me from dissolving into the fear that I am broken, not just my vagina and my bladder but some deep core of me that no one can ever touch.

Stress incontinence is what I have, Veronica tells me when I return for my next PT session, where she looks at my diary. This means that movement puts pressure, or stress, on my bladder, which causes me to leak urine.

As we're talking, I make the connection that motherhood puts a stress, an emotional pressure, on me that has caused my history to spill too. I'm interpreting everything with this filter now: motherhood + trauma. Recently when I reached for shampoo, I saw the descriptor *curl-defining*, and I couldn't read it without thinking, *trauma-defining*. *Motherhood is a trauma-defining agent.* Any small interaction can highlight, define, amplify my trauma unexpectedly.

People sometimes tell me about my baby: *You are his whole world.*

I smile and nod, but I swallow hard. I never want to be someone's whole world again.

In the bathroom I pull my labia to the side to take a peek at my tear with my sparkly red mirror. When I release my fingers, my lips close slowly but not fully. The doors remain cracked open. Maybe I gaze inside and search my body for reality and words because I want to know that I'm still here. I want to know how to become my own world while I also become a mother.

volcano

When I was a little girl, Dad drove me to beaches, state parks, and volleyball courts where he taught me to run the metal detector over the ground slowly. When the machine started beeping, we would slow down to trace the gray saucer over a cubic foot until the jumpy *beep beep* quickened into a solid *buzz*. We marked an X on the ground with a stick, got on our knees, and dug, breaking up clots of dirt between our fingers. A diamond tennis bracelet, a silver watch, a gold ring— what would we find? Though we sought precious metals, we knew that mostly we would excavate rusted bottle caps and perhaps a neat old coin if we were lucky.

We never found anything with great monetary value, but I remember feeling that the dark body of the earth held mysteries and possibility in the losses of those who had traveled before. It was trained in me: my determination to dig for what could be redeemed from the hard-packed dirt, to take a crusted old thing and rub it against my shirt. To chip away the sediment with my thumbnail until it shone.

On our last hunt when I was a teenager, we drove to the hospital where he worked, on orange Yazoo clay bordered by concrete that would soon be jackhammered for an even larger parking lot. The sun was setting and the air chilled toward winter, and even though I didn't really want to be there, I still believed that we could find treasure. I still left with dirt under my fingernails.

Three years into my relationship with J, I made an appointment with the college's counselor. Diana was a petite blond woman with a cheerful demeanor. I talked to her about my father's new marriage and my grandmother's aggressive breast cancer. What I remember saying about J is how much I loved it when he played guitar for me and I sang, mentioning offhand that he sometimes fell into depression or anxiety. I walked her around the edges of my romance story.

"But he's always there for me. He loves me so much," I told her. "He likes to cook me turkey burgers and tacos. He's sweet to his dog and his niece and nephew."

J went back to school for an associate's degree. I wanted him to want it for himself, but he insisted he did it for me. Still, it seemed to be working; his mood lifted as he left the bar kitchens he hated. He got excited about the innards of computers, electrical circuits, and microcontrollers. He built a pond on our patio and bought goldfish that grew bigger than an aquarium would ever allow. Soon there were frog eggs and tadpoles.

He had wanted me to prove myself to him, and I did. I cut off all ties with Taylor, with Steve, and with everyone from the Greece trip. I didn't return to the frat houses, and I didn't touch alcohol. I covered myself with more lies that I told my family about where I was sleeping and eating. I learned the shadowy routes across campus that would make it less likely for me to be seen, avoiding my friends' invitations and my professors' disappointed faces about the latest essay I owed them.

What I'm certain I didn't tell Diana is the way J had driven circles around the city threatening to kill himself until I agreed to move in with him. Or how J had laid his body on mine until my breath became a leak. How his anger water cycled into tears. How then I took him in my arms while he said, *Cathy, I'm so scared, Cathy, I'm so sorry, Cathy, I deserve to die.* How it didn't feel as if he was hurting me so much as I felt white-hot pain pouring out of him that he allowed me to see, private and tender, flaming. Almost holy to witness from the one I loved. If J's pain was bigger than my pain, rich-girl daddy issues, never punched, never hungry, never cancer cells eating a parent from the bones out, then I could hold him there, in all his vulnerability, where the occasional violence felt more like loving a person suffering than a person inflicting.

"Is the sex still good?" my friend Roxanne asked me with wide eyes when I told her I'd been with my boyfriend for three years. Her dorm room was dimly lit with strands of colorful lights.

"Yes," I said. Because I could reliably reach orgasm when I was on top. Even as I said it, though, I wondered if it was true. Strawberry-flavored lube was a tingly fascination on my tongue, but I felt little desire for J. I couldn't deny that my attraction had waned, but I kept reaching for the satisfaction of making love with the man who loved me.

That week when we stood in front of the mirror brushing our teeth, J said, "I'm a fatso. No wonder you're not attracted to me."

If I didn't respond in the right way, I knew it would turn into hours of insecurities that I wanted to leave him, that I wanted to be with someone else.

"Do you want to fuck him? You want to fuck him, don't you? Say it—you want to suck his cock. I guarantee you that he wants to fuck you." He smiled grotesquely with a snarled lip while he gyrated his hips. There was a whole cast of suspects: my best friend on the newspaper staff, my anthro professor, the dad of a pre-K student, a mandolin player I'd interviewed. J planted me in underground desires with them all. I was too trusting and too naive to see it, he said, but he knew. I swatted him away. It was hard to know where his humor's edges blurred into accusation. I shook my head and rolled my eyes, though internally I still flinched at this coarse packaging of my sexual pleasure. Aside from the fact that even in the privacy of my head, I'd never thought *I want to fuck him* about a single person or salivated over the idea of *sucking a cock*, I felt humiliated by the pairings he constructed.

What hammered into me was that if another man wanted me, I was in a lust dance with him whether I wanted him or not. That I could be both a seductress—a whore even—with her own hot agenda of fucking and sucking and that I could simultaneously be a naive girl lacking enough sexual appetite and awareness of her own to even recognize when a man desired me.

One time he found a CD in my car that was Sharpie'd to say *django reinhardt* by the mandolin player I'd interviewed and befriended, and he snapped it in half, as if the sharing of swing jazz was the first step toward fluid swapping. This gesture struck me as childish but expected in a story where I had been cast in the role of Hot, Young Girlfriend, and he was Jealous Boyfriend.

After J bent the disc in his hand until it cracked, I held its sharp fissures, the metallic layer fractured to the plastic substrate. It wasn't my body he broke in his hands, but my desire snapped in half. Pleasure was replaced piece by piece with placation. I learned to make the right noises and moves for the whole act to advance routinely, after which I could return to the futon, the next episode of *The Office*, and my homework.

I'm a fatso. No wonder you're not attracted to me.

So in our bathroom under the yellow fluorescence as we brushed teeth, I used the power that was available to me: my body. Clamping my teeth down on the toothbrush bristles, I let one hand reach toward his soft front. I traced my finger over his pants until something stronger awoke in him. Until I willed him into believing he was something more, the more I wanted him to be. I let my eyes meet his in the mirror, and the sparkle I summoned was possible only because I saw the reflection of my own face in the periphery. I focused my eyes on my own strength, how powerful to make him hard, to feel the dewdrop of his cock fall like a single tear.

On the bed my body felt empty, like a throat before it sings, before the muscles constrict to perform. I saw his brown-gray curls, the silver bridge of his glasses on his temple, the plastic window blinds. I could feel his fear of my leaving and my hand would receive it; and I would join it to my own fear of being caged. I looped my ankles around his and held tight, knowing that if he believed I wanted him closer, deeper, I'd get a little more free, at least for a few days. I squeezed his shoulder blades, his hips. My hair pulled stiff under my shoulders. The smell of cigarette ash holding all around me, sweeping against my skin, tiny fires that once glowed. My breath singing at his ear, rising, rising, then panting, airy song of my own determination to survive. The heat of my own breath echoing back at me; that's where my attention flared.

I'd lived in Jackson for ten years before I learned that our city was built on top of a volcano. My Intro to Geology teacher taught us about the local aquifers, the permeable ground of water-bearing rock and the zone of saturation. Then one day he mentioned the volcano beneath us. Its dome was only about a mile away, buried 2,900 feet under a circular, mirrored building known as the Coliseum. Growing up, I'd attended minor league hockey games there and glossed my lips for an Incubus concert. More recently, I'd served food there when thousands of evacuees sheltered after Hurricane Katrina. In all those years, I never knew a volcano was underneath us, dense igneous rock with a seventy-five-million-year gap of explosive activity. Though technically it was extinct, the volcano still emanated tightly wrapped waves of gravity that looked like a densely packed bull's-eye on a Mississippi Office of Geology gravity map my professor showed us.

On average, it takes seven attempts for a woman to leave a relationship of domestic violence. I had tried to break up with J three times. The last two times, it had quickly devolved into a hostage situation where he wouldn't let me leave and he threatened to kill himself. It was a gravity I didn't know how to pull away from. I didn't know the statistic at the time and still lacked words for the abusive reality of our relationship, but I had begun to feel the force of the two highly charged states within me constantly: staying and leaving.

Volcanoes can go quiet for thousands of years and then one day reawaken. That's the way I stayed, a cold and quiet mountain, a good girlfriend. Inside, plates were converging, and hot mantle rock crept upward. Fissures were forming, with molten rock melting deep within me. I could feel it rising again, the viscous liquid fire.

In the winter of my junior year, a fellow French student and newspaper writer named Meagan walked up to me at the salad bar. Meagan was equal parts intellectual and playful, as quick to say *Hey, Lil' Catherine* as she was to crack jokes about Jean-Paul Sartre. She had her life together in an age-appropriate way for a college student, as opposed to my squirrelly version of playing marriage with J.

"Hey, Lil' Catherine, so I have a crazy idea. Would you want to go to France together this summer? You have family there, right?" I didn't need to think about it. The *yes* came out of me as a full-body immersion, just as the *yes* for Greece had.

I knew that months of sulking were ahead of me from J, but by that point I'd built emotional scar tissue with less sensitive nerve endings. When he lectured me, I let my mind wander to the same distant place I'd learned to occupy during sex. That cold and quiet mountain.

In France, Meagan laughed me back to warmth. In markets we bought single apples that we ate immediately as we walked, and we drank wine from the bottle by the Seine. On trains, we noted that French men didn't look away politely, but rather, would sustain an intensity of eye contact that could be described only as *eye sex*. When the wind pressed our dresses between our thighs, we laughed and called it *vent de viol, rape wind*. At Nana Jojo's young friend's house, I stayed up until the early morning speaking French with his roommate Jean-Louis, a poet. Jean-Louis kissed me in the hallway between our bedrooms, but I told him, *Je ne peut pas—I can't,* and said good night. When we left, he gave me his hoodie for the train ride.

Once again I felt the clarity I'd had in Greece three years before: the feeling of being free. That I was twenty years old with many choices and possibilities ahead of me. The hard-packed dirt of the last three years began to break into clods, and glimpses of my shimmer returned.

After France, the charge toward leaving J gathered force in me.

Before a volcano erupts, there are warnings:
an increase in tremors and earthquakes, subtle swelling
of the ground surface, rises in the temperature and
changes in the chemistry of groundwater.

It was January of my senior year when I went to Hal and Mal's, a bar downtown, to hear a bluegrass band with my aunt Deborah. She asked if I wanted to split one beer with her, and I said yes. We drank it as we tapped our feet to fiddles and mandolins. When I came home, J leaned in close to smell my breath.

"You were drinking, weren't you?" For a moment I froze. My breath went still, my belly stiff. But then I drew in a new breath and let it out through my nostrils. Warmth began to rise through me, into my chest, into my throat, into my cheeks. My mouth opened.

"Yes, I had half of a beer. So what? I didn't do anything wrong."

We argued, a script so familiar that it was maddening, his words a confusion he threw over me. But this time I wouldn't let him bury me in his twisted version of who I was, what was right, and what I owed him. I didn't hold my breath. I let the air rush into my mouth, and I drank it wildly, along with the exhale of all that I'd been holding in. When his voice rose louder and louder, I didn't calm him with lies. I didn't say *I love you, I'm sorry, I was wrong.* I let him burn hot, and I showed no fear because I burned hot too.

"I would never want to have a baby with you," he said with the force of spit. "Thank God you won't be the mother of my children. You'll be a terrible mother. You don't deserve to be a mother. You'll abandon everyone who loves you."

I'm not sure if our dogs were in the room watching or if they were sleeping; I don't remember if we argued for one more hour or one more minute. What I remember is what his body did to my body when his words couldn't hold me down anymore.

The grip of his fingers on my arm.

The sound of his anger becoming unzipped into laughter, as if he could finally show me just how miserable the world was, a fact he'd always known but I still refused to believe.

He wanted to prove it to me, already hard, forcing himself into my mouth.

I pushed his hips back and said his name like a question, like a mother who sounds more angry than afraid when her child reaches for the hot pan.

The power he felt rising in me was what he reversed on me next, along with the Mace on my keychain.

My body went cold, like river water, while my mouth opened. My tears slid down my cheeks to the dead-end of my chest. My tongue was the only muscle I used to protect myself, and it went slick all down my throat.

Cretaceous rim of fire. Compaction and the drapery of sedi-mentary formations. Magmatic halo around Jackson.

In the morning, when the sun was still low, I left quietly for class as if nothing had happened the night before. *Rape.* For days I returned to the house and fake smiled and listened to guitar music and slept on the edge of the bed facing the wall, moving through the stale motions while everything under my skin shifted with terrifying heat for the breakaway. *Rape.* My skin could hardly contain me. My name felt strange on his tongue.

Geophysical unrest. Deep ocean trench. Rupture in the crust of a planetary mass that allows hot lava, volcanic ash, and gases to escape from a magma chamber below the surface.

J who never kills spiders. J singing with me in cars and stoops and parks and bedrooms and hallways. J playing shows in bars on Halloween, playing shows in Irish pubs, playing shows in grunge dungeons with red lights and brown plaid couches. J driving his Corolla past the cowboy boot shop by the fairgrounds with the 4-H stalls, while we hummed our jingle with a twang, saying *boots and boots and boots and more.* J with the restless legs that I rubbed in the night. J who ordered hamburgers plain, *Just the meat and the bun.* J driving me to the cypress swamp, to the Pearl River trail under the interstate, to haunted gravel roads with abandoned fridges and decomposing easy chairs. J saying, *I was lying in bed last night and a happy thought came to me . . . no, I probably shouldn't tell you.* J wanting to marry me. J wanting to die.

J driving me to his memaw's house where we deconstructed a beaver dam. J breathing slowly on my neck while he hummed three notes: *I love you.*

J forcing his penis in my mouth while I cried.

That was the only J I could allow myself to think about now. Because I needed to get far away from him, whether he lived or died. I didn't know how I would do it. But I needed to live, not die. Every bone cell, blood cell, and muscle cell told me: *Go.*

PART TWO

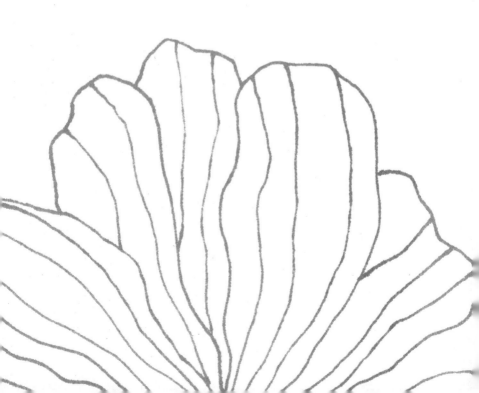

SILVER NITRATE

"Tell me what's been going on," Dr. S says, leaning forward and looking into my eyes with softness. After almost four months, I've already completed my last routine postpartum visit. I'm here for something different.

"Well, this is kind of embarrassing and strange," I begin, "but when I have gas, I feel it coming out of my vagina. I'm worried that there might be a tear between the rectum and vagina, a fistula." I use the word I learned in pelvic PT.

"Feeling gas coming out of the vagina is pretty common after a vaginal birth," Dr. S assures me, something about looser muscles and the travel of air. "Let's take a look."

I lie back on the table, the white paper crinkling underneath me. I lift my hips and scoot my butt to the end, positioning my feet in the heel-holds. A white sheet drapes across my thighs. Dr. S clicks on a bright light, shining directly into my grotto.

"You'll feel me touch your leg first," she says. Her latexed knuckle touches down on my inner thigh, butterfly landing on milkweed, and then touches one step closer to my pelvis. She knows I'm a survivor, and this is one of our safety measures.

The cold speculum lands at the introitus and then enters like a metal tongue. It expands inside me until I'm held open. Dr. S cranes her head to the side and lifts her chin as if peering around a corner. Her eyes narrow in focus before she stretches me open wider with her thumb and finger, ribboning pain along my labia scar. I exhale the rest of my breath.

"I'm sorry. I know this is uncomfortable," she says, keeping her gaze inside me. She's trained to keep the *oh-no* off her face, but she lingers like a bafflement, searching. "I see a lot of granulation inside here. I'm trying to get under the tissue to see the tear. It's extremely friable."

"Fry-able?"

"Yes, it's beefy red, more sensitive than regular tissue. It bleeds when I touch it." Her probing sweeps and titters inside me.

"What is the granulation?" I ask, my eyebrows tightening. In my mind: a cavern of crystals, big granules of sugar hanging from the ceiling.

"It's extra scar tissue," she explains, pausing to look at me. "It's kind of like overhealing. Your body responds to the wound by creating too much scar tissue. Do you want to take a look?"

I nod.

The nurse passes me a Caboodle-green mirror, the kind I've used to look at the back of my head after a haircut. But today I will use it to gaze into my tender, beefy vagina. I hold the mirror in my right hand and position it at my opening.

Seeing this internal view for the first time, speculum-wide, I try to orient myself to the vast fluff of glossy pink. It is so much lumpier than I thought, a cotton candy cloud land, not smooth like the view down my throat. Then I see it: a flap of tissue that looks to be about the size of a monarch caterpillar, attached to the valley of my birth wound.

Dr. S lifts the long flap with an oversized Q-tip and flops it from side to side.

"This is not normal vaginal tissue. It is very vascular tissue. See how it bleeds when I touch it?" She strokes the end of the cotton swab on the body of the scar, and the flesh blooms rose red. Like an optical illusion, like sorcery, blood conjured by the soft sweep of cotton.

I've felt like a weakling for still being limited by pain, for not being able to squat down to Guider's eye level without fearing my seams would bust open. My vagina's pulp has been sliding me secrets for months that something is wrong. I was right. Still, my thoughts slip under me as the flesh-locus appears in the mirror. I grab the first question I can reach.

"Is this why sex hurts so much now?" We've tried only once since birth, and the attempt had me grasping for words metallic and sharp. *Chicken wire. Cheese grater.* Lloyd barely moved inside me before slowly extracting himself with white-gloved precision.

"Absolutely. You can't even touch it without bleeding. Friction would be very painful." She pauses. "Are you sure your tear was second degree?"

"As far as I know, yes. That's what my midwife told me."

"Do you know what kind of sutures were used?"

I don't. I remember only the stick figure that Lydia drew on the paper towel, the tear going in two directions. Dr. S dresses her face with neutrality, but maybe she's holding something back in diplomacy. She slips the speculum out, pulls off her gloves, and offers her hand to help me sit up. I tuck the drape under my thighs, sweaty with tension.

"What caused this?" I ask, a cautious step toward mystery.

She explains that when vaginal and perineal tears are being repaired, everything is very swollen from birth. Sometimes when the edges of a tear are brought together to be sutured, *mucosa to mucosa*, an extra lip of tissue is created. That lip of tissue can become extra sensitive because tissue from the inside is now on the outside.

"All the healing is sent to that area, and it actually prevents the original wound from healing. A secondary wound is created." She pauses and waits for me to process.

I'm trying to not make poetry of it as she talks, but the words seem to communicate a greater truth than blood vessels and connective tissue. *Overhealing. Secondary wound.* I make myself stay in the physical realm to listen, my eyes like pollinators landing on the tissue box by the sink, the red sharps container in the corner, and the flashing tessellations of the computer screensaver, where they pick up my doctor's words and fertilize new questions in my mind.

She tells me what we must do: In order to allow the original birth wound to heal, the extra scar tissue must be killed. My sutures, designed to dissolve after two weeks, are still intact four months later underneath the hood of scars. No wonder I've felt the strain of seams inside me, as if standing for too long could split me open under the weight of my organs. Stitches still lace me together.

We'll use silver nitrate, a cauterizing agent, to kill the scar tissue "in hopes that the lack of blood supply to the area will cause the tissue to retract, die off, and fall off."

When Dr. S returns, she gathers her supplies on a rolling metal table and inserts the speculum again. There are four six-inch-long sticks of silver nitrate, shaded dark gray on the end like matchsticks. The nurse holds the metal clamp in place while Dr. S uses her right hand to grab the silver nitrate.

"You might feel some discomfort," she says and begins scratching the surface of the scar tissue with the stick's tip, like a grainy pencil made of acid. With a mirror, I watch my scar tissue fizzle from red to gray, from blood to cinders. Tingling, then stinging, then burning, like pepper oil rubbed in my membranes.

"It's responding really well to the silver nitrate," she says. The flesh surrenders and wilts into winter-gray knots. But soon I feel the fingers of heat branching in new directions, and the flames smolder deeper.

"The area around it is burning. It's spreading," I say.

"Vaseline, please," my doctor instructs the nurse, holding out her hand surgically.

With a Q-tip as long as a paintbrush, she rubs a gum-ball of oily protectant around the edges so the burning won't claim the surrounding tissue.

When it's over, I sit up and my vagina blazes beneath me, a wildfire.

"You might feel irritation and see some gray tissue passing in your underwear as it dies," she warns. A bath tonight will help soothe the tenderness. I'll probably need three more treatments to eradicate the scars. "What questions do you have for me?"

My eyes squint, and metallic nausea balloons my head. The Vaseline liquefies and trickles into my underwear.

"I feel like this is pretty obvious, but I shouldn't have sex, right?" I ask, realizing I ask a lot of questions about sex for someone who's had it only once in four months.

"Right. No sex for ten days. Were you to have sex, he would get a chemical burn on his penis." What I've just endured settles in me. The burning mounts and rises, a fire ladder.

"So . . . this is what I have? A chemical burn in my vagina?" She must see the question on my face: *Will I be okay?*

"The vagina is a very forgiving place—one of the most forgiving places on the body," she assures me with a gentle smile. "It's designed to stretch and tear and return to a healthy state. It's basically made to withstand trauma."

The vagina is a forgiving place.

Whatever I don't quite understand about my womanhood and my history begins gathering in this room, equal parts questions and answers. *Basically made to withstand trauma.* I know she means that birth is a trauma to the tissues, medically. Core truths of my female organs. But a more central understanding is beginning to open, like a seed cracked in half by a tender green shoot, before I know what flower or fruit it will become.

When I step out of the clinic, the sky opens bright and cloudless. The wind flicks a strand of hair into my mouth that I fish out with my fingers. The inside of my car is warm like a greenhouse, usually cozy against my cold winter cheeks. But when my body presses into the seat, my vagina becomes a fire-tempest licking upward. I lock the doors and unzip my puffy coat.

Something whirls in me, an updraft of anger. But I don't yet recognize it as anger because I've so rarely let myself sit with its hot bolts. I'm used to welding anger into sadness, a more palatable emotion for a girl and a woman to express. A safer feeling, nonthreatening.

I sit in the silence, key unturned in the ignition. I'm not ready to return home to four sticky hands palming my skin and a hungry mouth hunting my nipple. I can already feel the combustion swelling in me, my patience radiating thermal.

It is January 2019, a little more than a year after the #MeToo hashtags first went viral. Terms like *enthusiastic consent* and *toxic masculinity* have been swirling in the collective dialogue. Everyday, when I touch my phone, it lights up with red-carpet faces of women naming the assault and the men who inflicted. More than fifty-two weeks' worth of famous faces, and they keep coming. *Grab 'em by the pussy* still rattles in my head, tin cans dragged on concrete. New names and faces introduce themselves from this violent void and become new stars in my sky. A few days before Rowan was born, Brett Kavanaugh was appointed to the Supreme Court after a lengthy hearing that included vulnerable testimony from Dr. Christine Blasey Ford of alleged sexual assault in their teen years. I wouldn't let myself watch her right hand rise into the air, swearing to tell the whole truth, while I waited for birth to veer into me like a massive weather system, while I chanted *A sense of well-being fills my whole body*. I couldn't let the supreme chorus of violence closer.

My sadness is true, and it says: behold the plot line of the mother's vagina. Frictioned, stretched, torn, stitched, changed. My body, a flexible conduit. Penis in, baby out. *Vagina*, from the Latin, meaning *sheath, covering, husk*. A sheath is important because of how it exists in relation to the object that fills it. To be the hollow space that fills around a man's will and assertion—that was the assignment that no one told me to complete but I still studied.

The vagina is a forgiving place. Basically made to withstand trauma.

It echoes in me as I drive home, with the mood of a fever building heat, the body doing its job to fight the intruder and make a hostile environment for the pathogens.

It is January 29, 2019. Ten years ago on this day, I was preparing to escape my first romantic relationship. I don't do the math on the day my vagina is burned, but I don't need to. My body remembers the eruption.

After dinner, I excuse myself to the bathtub, where I gorge on a buffet of Google. *Granulation. Friable. Vascular. Second-degree tear. Mucosa.* I look at pictures of horse hooves adorned with flaming scar tissue like my own. I click through slides that differentiate between first- to fourth-degree childbirth tears, with diagrams and bullet points clustered on lecture hall blue.

Chemical burn. Cauterize. Silver nitrate. Silver nitrate sticks are used as a cauterizing agent, a technique of burning the skin or tissue so that it will stop bleeding, to prevent infection in a wound, or to kill hypergranulation, excessive scar tissue like my own. I learn silver nitrate was once called *lunar caustic* because ancient alchemists called silver *luna*, associating it with the moon. I soften into this angle. It sounds kind of magical, witchy even. Moon cycles, menstrual cycles, and the lunar caustic in my vagina. The first word I learned in French was *la lune* because Nana said it every time we saw the moon. The first sentence: *Je suis fatiguée. I am tired.*

When I click on silver nitrate on PubChem, a chemistry database of the National Institutes of Health, I see three warning pictograms shaped like red diamonds with black sketches: a flaming red fireball, hands under a faucet with zigzags sizzling above them, and a dead fish floating to the surface of wavy water. There are warnings:

- May intensify fire
- Causes severe skin burns and eye damage
- Very toxic to aquatic life, acute hazard, with long-lasting effects

I've avoided parabens in my shampoo and drunk filtered water only to have my most tender insides glazed with toxic, coral-killing sludge. I stay in the bathtub until the water goes lukewarm.

The abuse left no bruises. There is no police report, no restraining order. There were no swabs, no photos, no evidence. There is only my memory and my body.

When my anger wants to fight for me, when the mother in me rages for the girl I was, I can see the skeletal version upon which my story's skin drapes: A twenty-four-year-old man preys on a sixteen-year-old girl. Woos her, fucks her, coerces her, controls her, films her, ensnares her for four years with threats of suicide, rapes her, stalks her. That's the story. Forget the goddamn love story. Forget the camping and the rocky creek walks and the classical guitar. There is no love story here. The love story is a distraction from an epidemic of violence against women and the men who abuse. This is a story of a predator and a victim.

Sometimes I find myself saying *the breakup* and I correct myself—*my escape*. For years I used the digits of the day I broke away as the key to unlock all my passwords: 2-3-09.

I struggle to remember the exact date that Lloyd proposed to me, but I will never forget the day when I drove away from J's house for the last time, the day I tore free.

On the second day after the silver nitrate ignites me, I soak in the tub again, and a piece floats out. This one looks like a skinny strand of brain. Or like a coil of ground beef that rotted and fell from my womb. Strange, gray fruit. Not products of the violence, not medically, but physical markers of what I've survived—what I'm still surviving. I lift the alien, dead part of me with toilet paper and examine its color and texture with the same care as the blood-tinged mucus before birth, wondering, *What labor is ahead?* and saying, *It's time.*

hummingbird

I hadn't taken a class with Dr. Hopkins since freshman year, but our conversation stayed with me, pulsing with promise. *How would you feel if you broke up tomorrow?* *Relieved.* That's how I found myself back in his office, where a bookshelf full of philosophy and logic towered behind him. His bald head shone fluorescent, his eyes were steady behind his silver glasses, and his voice was level. I could hardly believe the words coming out of my mouth. *My car keys wrenched from me, my pepper spray in his hand, his fingers gripping my arm, his penis forced in my mouth.*

"Catherine, what happened to you is a form of rape," Dr. Hopkins told me. I nodded and swallowed. I hadn't used the word aloud. I had told no one.

"I can't break up with him in person. Would it be okay to send an email?" I asked. Breaking up in an email seemed like a weak move after four and a half years together.

"You don't owe him anything," Dr. Hopkins asserted. "You don't owe him a breakup or an explanation. What feels right to you?"

We decided I would come back the next day with a draft of an email. An email would provide time-stamped evidence if I needed to show it to the police later.

There are two seasons in Mississippi: summer and not summer. The only thing we can rely on is the heat. The rest of the year is a purgatory, trembling between cold and warm. The joints of the trees become visible, and the spider eggs nestle under piles of leaf litter, waiting for spring to be born. But we wander in the unknown, wondering if there will be snow this year or if a mosquito will skulk against our windowpane. Winter brings hot cocoa and chicken pot pie, a few good days for my warmest alpaca sweater, but these cheers dangle as lusts to be seized with our hands, not knowing how long they'll last or when they'll become artifices of a season that doesn't want us. We blow around this way until the heat returns.

It was early February, so it was not summer. In the library, I sat with a sheet of college-ruled paper and wrote.

> *J,*
>
> *I've been thinking about this for a long time and have decided we can't be together anymore. We need to break up. I don't think we're healthy for each other. We have very different ideas about the world, the kind of lifestyle we want, and our expectations of each other. We have had so many conversations in the past in which we have unsuccessfully tried to reconcile these differences, and it's obvious we will never share opinions on these things. I want to be happy, and I want you to be happy, and neither of us should have to give up our fundamental values for anyone. I still remember and value the good times we've had together, but I know*

*we are not compatible in many ways. You yourself have
said many times that you always knew this wouldn't work.
I have made my decision and am firm in my decision. I will
not change my mind, and I need and expect you to respect
my decision.*

*Nothing will be gained from any communication in the
future. Thus, I expect you to:*

- *Not call me*
- *Not come on campus*
- *Not try to contact me in any way*
- *Not come near me*

*Be aware that campus security will not let you onto
grounds. I wish you well, but there's no need to contact me
anymore.*

I returned to Dr. Hopkins's office, and we made a plan. The
air was woolly all around me, and I floated half in a dream.
The mist whited out the buildings and even my hands, but
a force of motion carried me forward in choreography my
muscles followed.

I woke up at J's house and stuffed only a few belongings in my
car, nothing that he could miss when scanning the room. I
kissed our rescue dog Zeke on the top of his bony head, swallowing hard, and rubbed Red's velvet ears. I shut my car door
and reversed, driving away from four years that streamed like
a watercolor behind me, with undefined edges and shapes
that morphed in the rearview, blurred by the violent ending.

In my dorm room, I opened my laptop and began typing
the email I'd drafted by hand. I sat on my twin bed, on the

blue and brown Scandinavian tree duvet I'd picked out when college had stretched like a freedom ahead. I felt far from that freedom now, far from the Summer of Love and the long-haired people holding hands and kissing in fields, far from the girl who wanted to be moonlight, starlight, sunshine, waterfall.

I typed J's email address, filled my belly with breath, and tapped the bright *send* symbol, which was the shape of a paper airplane. I imagined I was sending a paper airplane into fire.

After, my fingers couldn't find stillness. I combed my scalp, squeezed my lips, rubbed the corners of my eyes, and scratched the skin at my hairline. I waited for soundless eruption, for the smoke and the tremors, as if I could sense J reading my words and sending ripples of fury across the city. I wished I could hide in an underground vault with no windows, where he could never find me. Instead, I continued with the plan. I created a folder where his replies would automatically go, into a burned-out tree hollow where I didn't have to look. I opened my purple flip phone and blocked his number. I walked to my hall door, tore off my name my RA had decorated in peppy script, and crumpled the pink construction paper before burying it in the trash. He'd never been to my dorm room before, which was a comfort.

I knocked on my suitemates' door, connected by our bathroom. Together we were three variations of Katherine, Kathryn, and Catherine.

"If someone comes to the door looking for me, pretend you don't know me," I told them. "Lock the door. Call campus security. It's probably my ex-boyfriend who's not taking our breakup well."

Breakup was what I said; *escape* hadn't occurred to me yet and wouldn't for years. Still, fear seeped through me. I never thought he would rape me, but now I didn't know what he was capable of doing. A threat inside me pinched with the sharp notes of his voice and the quiver of his lip, even though he'd never said it aloud: *If I can't have you, nobody can.* With it came curiosities like how many liters of blood the human body holds and how much blood you can lose without dying. With it came flashes of his hands on the steering wheel while we plunged off the bluff into the dark goodbye of the Mississippi River. I pushed these thoughts from my mind.

Hummingbirds have long wings that can rotate 180 degrees, flitting backward and forward horizontally in a figure-eight motion. This allows them to create lift on both forward and backward wing strokes, generating quick changes in direction and speedy flight.

I flew across the sidewalks to the student center and rose up the stairs to the second floor to find the head of campus security. I'd interviewed John dozens of times about break-ins, frat party fights, and other breaches and hazards we reported in the college newspaper. He sat at his desk wearing khakis and a purple polo, his blond hair neatly trimmed around his temples, and his whole face a gleaming smile as he invited me in. My mouth felt thinly frozen as I told him about the threat to my safety.

"Catherine, we've talked a lot over the years. About some tough stuff too," John said. He had the eyes of a worried father; I had babysat his daughter before. "I've never seen you like this. You have tears in your eyes." I swallowed saliva that clung to my throat.

He gave me his cellphone number to put on speed dial. Later, back in my dorm, I would practice flipping my phone open and finding his name, like a quick draw in a duel. I would send him a photo of J to give to the security guards.

Relief began to melt into me, even as my hands shook. For years I'd kept the relationship separate and hidden, like compacted strata, while above ground I operated as a functional, dual-major college student, even working my way up to editor-in-chief of the college newspaper. To become a riverbank of muddy mess, of trampled moss and dog piss, was part of what I willed myself toward. That was the way toward safety and morning light.

Shaky but resolute, I went back to Dr. Hopkins's office and looked into his eyes again. I told him I had done it. I sent the email. Again, his voice came out level and calm.

"Don't go anywhere alone for three months," he advised, a length of time that he didn't back up with statistics but that I absorbed with the trust of a child chewing a multivitamin. "If he tries to contact you after three months, add another month. Keep doing this until he stops."

"Do you think it's a good idea for me to tell people what happened?" I asked.

"Tell as many people as you feel comfortable telling," he said. "Tell everyone."

I hadn't yet read that leaving an abuser is the most dangerous time for a victim of domestic violence, but my body knew. I became aware of my blood pushing inside my veins. I became aware of my chest filling with my breath, the wonder and fragility of my body alive. When I sat on the toilet, I found words quietly floating from me, like dust shaken from a garment. *I am wiping my butt, and I am nobody's girlfriend.* When I stepped out of the shower: *I am drying my skin, and I am free.*

I remembered being twelve years old and riding in the back seat as I looked at my hands in my lap and tried to imagine they were someone else's hands. There was a dial I could slowly turn in my vision until my familiar hands could become othered, outside me. Strange fingernails, strange knuckle lines, strange palm shape.

Now I looked down at my hands, and I turned the dial the other direction, toward recognizing my fingers as my own, with the awareness that they would never make contact with J's skin again. This both comforted and unsettled me. We had spent four and a half years together, and despite all the pain, I still loved him. My hands in those years were always traveling back and forth in contact with his. Next to my hands were his hands, making chords on the guitar neck and typing on his keyboard and lighting cigarettes and petting our dogs.

If I had to draw a map of the last four years to illustrate my movement day to day, the map's constant point of return would be J's hands. To class and back. To the coffee shop and back. To the library and back. To the newspaper office and back. To the airport and back. And back, again and again, to his hands.

I looked down at my hands for the first time since I was seventeen knowing there was no *back*. There was only me, everywhere else, forward.

The night I sent the email, fear began to pour into me. Lying in my bed pushed up to the cold window, I couldn't shake the churning sense of being watched. My heart thrummed in my neck, where I pushed my thumb pad into the soft hollow of skin where my pulse thrashed like a small bird. I couldn't vanish the thought of crime scene tape and the bleed of police sirens. I imagined J waiting for me outside. J streaming in with a *Thank you* behind an innocent card swipe at the stairwell. J unfastening the lock at my door.

I felt as if I was overreacting, losing it, as if my brain was glitching. If J could see my thoughts, he would be horrified to know the fears that pinned my limbs. He would say, *Cathy, how could you think I would ever do that to you?*

In the middle of our relationship, he began crafting short horror films, sometimes with his brother and sometimes with friends. One involved zombie gore makeup, and another involved remote train tracks. In one of them, I drove my car down a country road a dozen times at night in order to get the shot he wanted of a woman returning home to her trailer, where she would be killed. J tried to talk me into playing the woman in the shower, a scene that would end with strangulation. I refused. But he described his vision so many times with a hardened candy smile on his face that the scene existed in my head. I could see myself on-screen, crying and unable to cry out for help, my long wet hair ending across the fig brown of my nipples. Now it loomed as a disturbing fantasy that he never got to complete. Sometimes while driving or showering, I realized the scene was playing on a loop in my head. I died over and over while he watched.

It occurs to me now that maybe he did make the movie that he wanted. I was the actor, and I was the audience. Then and still.

As I lay in bed, I turned my imagination instead to the riddle of the protective layers around me: walls, doors, fences, brass locks. I was the small nut hidden at the center. I nestled like a tiny, acorn-bodied doll in a twin bed, within a room, within a larger room, within a floor, within a building, within a series of buildings, within a tall metal fence. Between J and me all these layers thickened. This helped my body soften into the reassurance of my blanket around me.

Still, I decided I would call Dad the next day and tell him I needed to talk with him, that J and I broke up and I had concerns. I wouldn't tell him the whole truth, but I would tell him enough to activate his force field of protection. Maybe I would even stay at his house for a few nights. J wouldn't dare confront me or hurt me there. He would meet certain devastation.

The hospital where Dad worked was visible from my campus, so it was easy for him to meet me for lunch the next day. I met him in the campus parking lot, and as I walked next to him, he squeezed my neck affectionately. I was nervous to share any part of my rivermelt truth, to cast myself as the daughter in distress, and it was also hard to feel how much I needed him. My organs squished liquid warm and pierceable, but next to Dad, I took on the posture of a person who believed she would go on living. Dad has hunted wild boar and fought robbers off his gold chain in a dark Denny's parking lot. Dad's presence is a glint of metal, a white-knuckled grip on a leather knife handle, a thick, hairy man arm. Next to him, I could summon my iron core of survival. I rubbed my own hairy arm.

As we walked downstairs into the soup and sandwich café, suddenly I saw the last thing I wanted to see. Curly hair and glasses. J was walking toward us, past the mailboxes and the bookstore down the hall. I nudged Dad's arm to say, *There's J. Please help.* Dad went cool and tall. I don't remember what he said, but he didn't have to make threats or raise his voice. He became a river fjord, a steep wall of rock between J and me, saying something simple about eating lunch with his daughter. They said a few phrases back and forth, calm, dry words I don't remember. I was barely a drift of breath. J left, red-eyed and polite. I could see the pain leaking from him, the reservoir held thinly behind that leak, but I let the trickle stream as he walked away.

All the protection and overprotection from my father that I'd been evading for years I now wanted to wrap around me like a chainmail swaddle. I packed a bag and slept at his house for two weeks. I didn't tell him much about J because I didn't want him to hurt him. But I stayed safe, as I suspected I would under his roof. I slept in the guest room because my old room was being decorated as a nursery for a baby with his new wife.

On cold nights, the ruby-throated hummingbirds enter a temporary state of torpor in order to conserve energy. Lowering their body temperature and heart rate, they edge a controlled hypothermia. The next morning, the hummingbird needs only a few minutes to revive its body temperature to normal.

Hey, are you ready to go to the Caf? I texted my friends at dinnertime once I returned to campus. There were about ten people whom I'd told some version of: *I broke up with my boyfriend. It got intense. I'm kinda worried he might be violent. Probably nothing. Can I call you if I need someone to walk with me?* While we walked, even as we laughed about the *SNL* song "Jizz in My Pants," my eyes mapped the territory in every direction, with the blood sense of prey. When my phone vibrated, I quickly pressed the silence button while my heart flapped into my throat.

After a few weeks, once I was inside a safe place with a locked door, there was little space for sorrow. In the last semester of college everything was last hurrah, senior wine tasting, comprehensive exam prep, and resumé bullet points. Something was ending for all of us, but the chorus spirit was commencement.

Small fragments of normal college life winged me forward: Eating pizza on Valentine's Day with my single ladies, all of us in black dresses with ecstatic cleavage and voluptuous smiles. Giggling through Meagan's hijinks of hiding a creepy baby doll arm in her roommates' cereal box and underwear drawers. Charter busing to New Orleans for my gay friend's fraternity ball, powdering our noses with midnight beignet sugar. Riding around Jackson in a limo with glow sticks, slapping lacy thonged asses for a twenty-first birthday. Walking through Belhaven on a Sunday morning with a mouth full of espresso and Simone de Beauvoir.

I was the prodigal friend suddenly returned home. I hadn't known if I would be welcomed back into the flock, but I was, fully, more than I felt I deserved after pushing away my best friends for a couple years. Never far from my mind were other women who needed to escape violence but who didn't have a fully furnished dorm room, a father's bank account, and a community holding them. I wanted to give more than thanks. I wanted to live. The word *victim* had no space in my consciousness. Instead, the word that flew from me was *resurrection*, returned from the dead. Brilliant red feathers fruited my throat like an offering to the divine that allowed me to rise, to flap, and to hover in the garden that always grew my feast. Even my shadow seemed to flush warm beneath me, sweet surprise of motion that showed I was alive. My hunger was huge, and the taste of my tongue and the sugar were the same.

OVERHEALER

"February's hard for you, isn't it?" my friend Natalie asks me. I'm sitting on the couch looking out the living room window, oak branches like bony fingers.

February's the month when I escaped J, which Natalie knows but she doesn't say it. My kids call her Aunt Fairy because she's their *fairy godmother*, but she was Lloyd's friend first; they studied abroad in Costa Rica together. She's known me since the first months I got free, since I fell in love with Lloyd.

The kids are pulling on me to get off the phone, and the wind of impatience is picking up force in me, so I say, *Goodbye, see you soon, feel better, let me know if you need anything.* It's the coldest and darkest month in Mississippi, when plans get canceled because someone's kid has a fever or vomited in the night. It's crushing when I try to do a good thing for myself—getting out of the house, looking in the eyes of a friend—but it falls apart. A maddening isolation can set in, like during the years of abuse when my friends were only a few miles away but felt unreachable.

I squat on the floor to pull Rowan's pants on him. Guider runs up behind me and tries to climb on my back. His hands wrap around my neck, the weight in his fingers pressing into my esophagus. I almost topple backward. My heart beats faster, thorns growing.

I am the adult, I remind myself. *He is the child. I have the power.*

"Please stop. I don't want you on my back right now," I manage to say.

But his fingers wrap around my neck again, and he is laughing. A game, a test. The thorns grow, wrapping around my chest, where my breath freezes. My first impulse is to tear his fingers off my neck and shove him off my body with all my force. The promise of that relief hisses. But I pause. I get a flash of that ending: his back hitting the wood floor, a thread of spit knitting his cry, the glossy terror in his eyes as he beholds his mother.

"No. That hurts me," I say firmly. "I asked you to stop."

"Mama, no. You love me." His lips plump into a frown.

"Stop saying that."

I remind myself: *He's two years old. He's learning to use words. He's not manipulating me. Love is not a device of control in our house.*

"I do love you. Very much," I tell him, halting my hands with the bunched-up pants in order to focus on his eyes. "Listen. This is important. Even when you love someone, you get to decide how you want your body touched. I do too."

The other day I stood up for him in this way at Nana's house. *Look, he gave me a hug. He's a good boy*, Nana Jojo cajoled Guider. He'd wriggled out of her hug while his god-brother went into one willingly. *I'll be so sad if you don't hug me*, she pouted.

Good boys don't have to hug, I told him loudly enough for everyone to hear. *Good boys are allowed to not hug. They can say* no *if they don't want to be hugged. That's good, too.*

Now I stand up and carry Rowan, in only his diaper, to the bathroom.

The drive to the gynecologist's office takes thirty minutes. Two weeks have passed, and it's time for my second treatment with silver nitrate.

Undress, gown, *knock knock* at the door, feet in the stirrups, and the spotlight's inside me. Dr. S is pleased to see that the scars have reduced by about 25 percent. My body is cooperating with the healing intervention.

"I'm going to need three silver nitrate sticks, Q-tips, Vaseline, and gauze," Dr. S tells the nurse. My center spreads open once more, revealing the middle of my middles, the core of my core. She begins the controlled burn, and I watch in the mirror. It doesn't take long this time; it already feels routine, although an image flashes in my head of a cigarette pressed into skin and singeing the flesh black.

As my tissues wilt and burn, I do not feel separate from other truths that bring gratitude:

I have free childcare once a week, sometimes twice, so that I can help my body heal.

I have a reliable car to drive to the clinic and to physical therapy, enough money for gas.

I have the emotional support from loved ones and therapy to build my capacity to seek out help—first, to know that I deserve it.

"Do you see this kind of growth often?" I ask when it's over and I'm sitting up. She shakes her head no. I still wonder if my midwife did something wrong, but I'm not ready to say it. I don't have space to process the possibility of harm, not while changing my panty liners twice a day and clinging to the sweetness of Rowan learning to roll over while Guider mirrors him by rolling across the nursery rug. I need to leave here and be a present mother, not a woman splayed on an emotional stretcher.

"This is the first time I've seen hypergranulation like this in my eighteen years of practice," she says. She's seen overgrowth of scar tissue in hysterectomy patients before, at the cuff of the uterus, but never inside the vagina from a birth injury. Not to this extent.

I nod, caught between the sobering reality of my body's rare condition and some twisted satisfaction that I am an extraordinary case. It lands like permission to feel how huge this wound seems, how confusing and tangled with my past history.

Dr. S wants to know if I've had scarring issues before, like keloids. I mention the stout raised scar over my heart, where a monitor was implanted a few years ago for the electrical issue in my heart. Some bodies simply respond to the natural healing process with an aggressive growth of scar tissue, she says. A minor burn, abrasion, mole removal, or mosquito bite can turn into a scar much larger than the original wound.

Am I a body, a person, who overresponds to wounds, whether emotional or physical? Have I overhealed emotionally too? Have I created too much scar tissue in response to the wounds of abuse, and is that armored coating actually hurting me rather than protecting me?

Surely there are limits to turning my physiological healing into a master class in how I heal emotional wounds. But

I want more. I move closer to this fire like an animal seeking warmth.

With the heat of the silver nitrate inside me, I return to the house queasy. My head radiates with dull ache. *Cut off the scars' blood supply. Tell your body its healing is whack*, my mind buzzes. With each burning, we are getting closer to the base of the wound, the place where I tore.

I lie on my side in bed nursing the baby. My belly pools in a soft pad in front of me, a big puddle of flesh.

"Mommy, what's in your bellie?" Guider asks me. "Is brother in your bellie?"

"Oh, nothing's in my belly," I say. "That's just fat and skin." He's more used to seeing his daddy shirtless, who couldn't pinch three letters' worth of fat if he tried. My weight is less than driftwood these days, though, a story that mattered before but is now the least interesting thing about my body. Aside from the fire in my underwear, nausea hangs around my neck like a feeding trough this afternoon. Side effect of the silver nitrate, I guess.

You will survive this. It's not cancer; it's not one year left to live, I tell myself. Don't be the Martyr Mother. Don't be the walk-on-eggshells mother. Don't be the catastrophe mother.

At the same time, I push against this self-criticism. Our culture is quick to find a way to blame and shame the mother. That culture lives inside me.

The internet is full of opinions on each faction of motherhood, stories that sound like the working mom and the stay-at-home mom; the breastfeeding mom, the formula mom, and the pumping mom; the natural birth mom, the cesarean mom, and the epidural mom; the cry-it-out mom and the attachment parenting mom; the organic homemade puree mom and the red dye 40 mom; the hot mess mom and the helicopter mom. There are many tidy ways to catalog a mother. I don't want to create a tidy new label called the Survivor Mother, but I want us to revere the complexity of our histories and our decisions.

The vagina is a forgiving place. The trauma of a mother's body happens not just to an individual but to a whole family, a whole community.

As I lie in bed with the nausea and the pain, I hear Mister Rogers's red-sweatered voice say, "Anything that is human is mentionable, and anything that is mentionable can be more manageable."

When I stand up from my chair, my vagina is a heavy undertow, a drag below me. I can't do anything without being aware of it. Similarly, not a day goes by that I don't think about J. An awareness in perpetuity.

I try to talk about the hypergranulation and the silver nitrate with close friends and family, but I can't communicate exactly what is happening. Their faces screw into pain at the pairing of *vagina* and *chemical burn*. My words stay in the clinical realm. There is a short in the fuses that keeps me from communicating the significance of what's happening, the story you wouldn't see in the clinical notes.

Feminist critic Jacqueline Rose writes about "violence's encroachment on the inner life of the victim." In *On Violence and On Violence Against Women*, she says: "Harassment is always a sexual demand, but it also carries a more sinister and pathetic injunction: 'You will think about me.'"

You will think about me. You will think about me when you are making love to your husband, when you are gazing into your baby's eyes, when you are looking at your body in the mirror. You will think about me.

"There have been times when I felt like I forgave him," I told my therapist, Kristen, the year after Guider was born and the memories of the sexual and psychological abuse flooded me. "But then later I felt angry again."

"That's okay," she said. "Sometimes we put stuff down and find we need to pick up the story again like a stone and carry it for awhile so we can understand something new about it."

The scars make my vagina produce more discharge. Is it weeping? Is it salivating? Maybe it is pouring out, telling its story.

I will let it. I'm ready to understand something new.

In daylight I open the hall closet and find the boot box that holds my old journals. Inside is my leather journal wrapped in a brown cord. I flip through the pages. There's a bumper sticker that says READ A FUCKING BOOK from anti-establishment.com. There's an Ani DiFranco lyric about capitalism being the devil's wet dream, Keith Haring postcards of yellow stick figures holding hands, and photos I took along the Pacific Coast Highway. Then I find the entries from the summer I met J. I start reading.

In my memory, on the night I met him, I scribbled in my journal, *I've met a boy.*

But today I find different words.

I've attracted a boy.

Red blood pulses faster. I'm startled by the agency of it. *Attracted.* My voice comes off the page with power. It doesn't match the story I've been playing in my head for years: victim and predator. And it's one coy sentence mentioned offhand at the end of two pages about the magic of that night, the music, the conversations. The *boy* is nameless, faceless, marginal.

He is like a big teddy bear, I wrote weeks later, *and our physicality centers around cuddling and jokes, so soft and slow that it feels feminine.*

I said that he wanted to hide the stretch marks on his belly and hips, but I caressed them. *They're yours, and I love you*, I said, lifting his black T-shirt to lay my lips there.

The more I read, the more I can't take my eyes off her, who I was at sixteen and seventeen. I expected to shake my head at her and think, *How stupid.* But I meet an introspective young woman who makes a lot of sense. She's insightful and fierce, with eyes open as she contemplates how to love a boyfriend and honor herself at the same time. I'd be proud if she were my daughter.

For years, I thought I was blindsided by J's behavior, but now I see that even in the first months of our relationship, I was questioning times when he was inconsistent, self-centered, and even cruel. I see my part in the beginning of our enmeshment. And I saw it back then too.

For some reason, when I am with him, I feel like a ditzy bimbo and a conceited bitch a lot of the time, which concerns me. Aren't people you love supposed to make you feel like your best self, not your worst?

*

Is this what first love is all about? I want to please J, to be forgiving, to play out his fantasies, and be his dream girl but sometimes I wonder if the only reason I'm doing all this

*is because he's my first love and I don't know any better. I
wonder if I will look back at this and think about how naive
I am to want to please him so much.*

*

*I don't write anymore, read anymore, or spend time alone.
I want to write a poem, but I feel like I've forgotten how. Is
this a natural love occurrence—the whole "me" to "we"
thing? I'm moody and feel like I can't socialize anymore.
I don't blame J for anything but surely he has influenced
me. Nana and Mom are scared of how close I am to J.
Sometimes it scares me, too, because I have forgotten a lot
of things about myself that I used to think I knew. Everything feels so hazy now. It's not fair to blame J; it's not his
fault that I've soaked up his mannerisms, interests, and
way of life. I just need to become my own person again
and to have a life separate from him.*

*

*If I leave for college, it's not in pursuit of love, to find another
boyfriend. If I leave, it will be so I can grow as an independent being and focus on myself.*

I wrote about the night when I cried on the phone with
him after I got college acceptance letters from schools in
Portland and California.

"Imagine how much you'll cry when you leave for Portland," he said.

"I haven't made up my mind yet," I told him.

"I know you're leaving," he said, defeated. "The forces
don't want me to be happy. But when Carole's husband and
your husband beat you later in life, at least I will have the satisfaction of knowing that you're thinking about how J always
treated you right."

My private response in my journal:

Isn't that twisted?

I had all these intentions and doubts, and still I stayed in Mississippi instead of leaving for college? How could I have decided to stay even with all that awareness?

Now that I'm a mother, I also grieve that I didn't share my concerns with my mother, my grandmother, or my aunt. I gave myself the job of holding everyone else's sorrows without allowing an adult who loved me a chance to guide or protect me.

Another inner voice comes in to say: *You couldn't have known how dangerous it would get. You can't blame yourself for what you didn't know. You were used to taking care of yourself emotionally.*

When I meet the girl I was and listen to her, really listen to her, I can understand her. I can believe her. I can trust her. I can love her. I can forgive her.

Maybe my body has been hanging onto the wound because I can't leave her behind. Like a mother, I've been waiting for her to return home, where I run my fingers down the length of her inky hair and she loosens her chest into my hug. Her cheekbone rests into my heart.

I read my journals late into the winter night while my children's mouths gape in bed. The next morning I read them again while I drink my coffee in bed; she wakes up next to me.

In pelvic PT, I lie on a mat on the floor while Veronica runs her hands along my lower abdomen to palpate my fascia.

"Feel this? It feels like webbing," she says. "That's scar tissue from your C-section." She slides her fingers in a U-shape around my belly button. The scars cover my whole belly like a fishing net with clusters of thick knots, pulling on my pelvic muscles and ligaments and causing restriction in the whole system.

"They will melt under your fingers like butter," Veronica says, teaching me how to massage the scars to loosen them, layer by layer. "If you press too hard, it can make the scars thicken."

The touch is so light that it's hard to believe it can heal anything. T-shirt lifted, I place my fingers as if to kiss the scars and say, *They're yours, and I love you.*

flaming azalea

Open air, open view. The center of campus dipped into the Bowl, a lush, grassy slope flanked by gnarly oaks and pink flame azaleas. On spring days like this one, Frisbees flew, fingers arched on guitars, and lovers pressed their bellies on blankets where book spines loosened. You lingered here if you wanted to be fed by the day's last light across talk of foreign films and ancient fertility nudes like the curvy Venus of Willendorf.

I was alone but reasonably safe, not somewhere I could be pulled into the passenger seat of J's Corolla. Here I could scream for help and be spotted immediately by college athletes on their way to dinner. These were calculations I made now.

When my heart wasn't beating so fast it felt like a hum, my relationship with J blurred into a crazy blip of college life. College had included no hard drugs, no STDs, no one-night stands, no arrests, no pregnancies, not even a failed class or a friend holding my hair while I vomited. This was my crazy college thing. But *my thing* felt very old, like wrinkled breasts in a pilling nightgown, as if I'd traded my youth to fall asleep on complaining bedsheets, in the hollow trance of lullabies that now felt like lies.

There were not yet widespread conversations with words like *gaslighting*, *toxic masculinity*, and *boundaries*, and Instagram would not be invented for more than a year, much longer for slide swipes of self-help flora. What I had was Virginia Woolf writing "to love makes one solitary" and the recognition of how much of me—the part I called *love*—had existed in a solitary place for my college years. I had Gothic lit, with the honorable Dr. Jekyll transforming out of the public eye into the violent and cruel Mr. Hyde, evoking my first impressions of J as sweet and shy, a teddy bear, and how, by the end, he would laugh while he forced his body inside my mouth. I had Mary Shelley's *Frankenstein*, with the creation of a sentient monster who repulses his creator, and the realization that J vivisected me into the parts he wanted and the parts he didn't. I had the epic fragments of *The Waste Land* by T. S. Eliot, with lines that echoed through me: "What are the roots that clutch, what branches grow / Out of this stony rubbish?"

I wasn't sure what could grow out of the rubble of my first love, but I'd search for the roots that survived the ruins.

I'd never played beer pong before. The ball, buoyant in my fingers, left my hand with a surprising amount of control and traveled a smooth arc through the air before plopping into the frothy beer. On the other side of the table was a boy in a shamrock blazer with gold buttons. Lloyd, a fellow English major, had asked me on a date the year before. I told him I had a boyfriend, but I also said, *Let's keep circulating,* because I liked being around him.

He was whole-grain wholesome, fed on his mama's chicken and rice casseroles and honey-glazed carrots, church suppers on Wednesday nights. But he was also delightfully weird, not a square but a wandering squiggle. A fellow of existential joy, he was playful enough in his gender to paint his fingernails and to craft his own skirt out of newspaper. I'd never met anyone like him. He'd written me a sonnet that he hand-delivered. Lloyd's crush on me had become a staff joke at the newspaper, where I stood at the whiteboard to field the week's article ideas while he perched with a gaze of adoration.

Tonight his eyes danced with his eyebrows, and his arms flowed in electric flourishes at the Ping-Pong table. He cheered as I landed shot after shot while he lost. Warmth rose in my cheeks with my smile. Here was a guy who wasn't intimidated by a woman's power but drawn to it. I wasn't looking for someone to couple with, but if there was joy to experience, I would welcome it.

J's voice was a pinched presence in my head, railing about the cheap beer, the frat house, the boy in the blazer who just wanted to fuck me, how it was all so stupid. But my life wasn't his feast any longer, and what I tasted, I wanted to taste for myself.

After Ping-Pong, Lloyd danced near me, windmilling his arms, dropping into sudden squats, and bouncing back up like a pogo stick before kicking high in the air. I turned and danced toward his joy.

Back in my dorm the next morning, I looked at my phone and saw a voicemail from J's mom. A jolt of panic radiated that maybe J had killed himself as he'd repeatedly threatened if I left. The next jolt was that J's voice might be in the message since I'd blocked his number. I didn't want to hear him raging, pleading, boy-crumbling—whatever version might be waiting for me. I didn't know what his mom might want to say, but she liked me in the way that a mother does when her son finds a nice girl he wants to marry. I'd enjoyed many dinners of her Frito pie.

I took a deep breath and pressed play.

It was her Velveeta-smooth voice, her melty Southern vowels.

"Catherine, J told me what happened. I'm so sorry. He feels just terrible about it. He's having a really hard time. I know you don't want to talk to him, but will you let me know that you forgive him? I don't know how else he'll move on."

J and I hadn't talked about what happened that night, what he did to me, and I wasn't sure how he remembered it. But from the pain in her voice, maybe he understood that he'd crossed a new, sickening line. He was probably crying in his mama's arms now instead of mine. Did he tell his mother that he sexually assaulted me, raped me, forced his penis in my mouth?

I *did* want him to move on—make music, play RPG video games, boil ramen, and accept that all of this would happen without me. I wanted him to leave me alone, forget about me, trash-talk me as another crazy whore girlfriend, whatever. I even hoped he would go on to have a good life, which, depending on the minute, made me feel either weak or like a creature of invincible light.

But let his mom know that I forgave him? This I could not do.

I could still hardly grasp what had happened.

Sometimes when I was alone in my room in the middle of writing an essay, I found myself Googling *definition of rape.* My eyes traveled across the search results on my laptop, confirming what was true over and over. Phrase by phrase, I broke it down.

Penetration, no matter how slight,
of the vagina or anus
with any body part or object,
or oral penetration by a sex organ of another person,
without the consent of the victim.

So much of my life with J over the past four years felt murky, but this definition was crisp. *Oral penetration by a sex organ. Without the consent of the victim.* I turned to it whenever the dust film of confusion adhered. There were no cotton swabs in my mouth at the hospital, no panties in a zip-tight bag, no photos of evidence. All I had was this definition.

Forgive him, his mother was asking? For years I forgave and forgave and forgave. All I did was forgive. I prioritized his pain and minimized my own. Now I was trying to thicken the barrier between us, to not tune into the twist of his pain shredding my belly and forgetting me into forgiveness. Some hours I felt cruel for ending the relationship in an email, cutting off contact without warning, metal slam of guillotine on a long-term relationship. But survival in me said, *Remember. Remember what he did.*

In one way, it was over, but in another way, it wasn't. I was still surviving him, trying to wrench myself free. Recently I'd been out for coffee with friends, and J showed up, stiff and buzzed with adrenaline. Though my friends had never met him, they scanned my face and his crazy eyes and knew.

J stood behind my friend's car so we couldn't leave. My heart pounded, and I was embarrassed. I didn't want to put anyone in the position of protecting me and maybe getting hurt; my friend Kyle tried to convince J to move out of the way. After the mention of calling the police, we were able to leave.

You can't forgive what you're still surviving. My most pressing goals were: stay alive, don't get sucked back into relationship with J, and return to myself. Other goals included: pass comps, graduate, and find a job. More goals: be a good friend, have fun and feel young, and find new songs to sing.

Forgiveness was a distant blossom coiled in the future, its mother seed not yet planted, not yet ripened inside a purple flower blossoming this season. It was several generations of seeds ahead, sleeping in rich roots, buried in soft soil, something that would grow with me, I hoped.

I had no sense yet of the magnitude that this rape and this relationship would have in my life. I had more questions than I cared to map, including: *How will I ever share myself fully again? When will I be interested in sex? Should I stay on birth control? Will he use the sex tape to punish me? Are my passwords strong enough?*

There were no simple answers, but I knew forgiveness wouldn't slide through me like a hand with a knife, pleading, *You could fix this! You could save him!*

My fingers did what they knew to do next. They blocked J's mother's number.

Wisteria, azalea, and dogwood held hands like best friends across fences, singing welcome songs to spring. I wanted to curl at their feet, in their sunlight, and let their pollen birth me from their trembling bodies. Forget about root rot, leaf loss, branch dieback, and wilting. Tell me not of canker, crown rot, and powdery mildew. Whorl me to the tips of my branches. Cluster me in trumpets of scarlet, apricot, and candle yellow. I wasn't born to hide.

My mom sent me a care package with cream-filled chocolate eggs. Over the phone I'd told her about the breakup, but I shared only the tightly knotted version of the story. She sighed in relief that I finally disentangled myself from a man who wasn't adventurous enough to try escargot at our Christmas table. I couldn't bear to take this happy moment from her and convert it into horror. I needed this happy moment, too, her cheering for me and my new freedom, not grieving over a violated daughter.

When I walked up to the library desk, I saw Lloyd sitting at the helm, where he checked out books. Our smiles preceded us. I handed him a cream-filled egg, and he unwrapped the bright green aluminum and popped the whole thing in his mouth. I gasped at his devouring.

"How do *you* eat it?" he asked.

"I take a bite or two and wrap up the rest for later." I unwrapped the chocolate egg I'd already nibbled to show him before returning it to my pocket. The idea of savoring a single sweet over multiple episodes astounded him. Later he would tell me, "I'd never met anyone who savored life so slowly and sumptuously, outside of a fine-dining restaurant, just in day-to-day life." When I saw it on his face, I felt joy was at my core, always whole like the moon.

Since the Ping-Pong night, we'd gone on a late-night Waffle House outing with one of my best friends, Sophia, who read poetry aloud with me and let herself laugh so hard that she drooled. We'd also taken a Saturday morning farmers market excursion with Lil' Meagan. As we drove away from the market, Lloyd said, "I'd like to dance with you and the ghosts over there," pointing to the concrete loading docks with rusted canopies. I laughed at him, but I liked his shameless honesty, how his lips matched his heart.

Recently I'd sat directly behind him in a dark classroom watching an Edward II film for our Elizabethan history plays class. The back of his neck kept tugging my attention away from the screen. Even in the dark, I could sense the warmth of his tan, goldened from hours running on Jackson's potholed streets. Two small moles bordered his T-shirt's neckline. I didn't need to touch his skin to notice the fuzzy smoothness. But for the first time I considered that I might like that. The curve of his shoulders under his T-shirt suggested muscle, not showy muscle but useful muscle built from the love of a body moving. I knew that he woke up at 7 a.m. to run no matter how late he'd stayed up the night before. He held himself tall, alert with curiosity, as if the world was asking him a question and he was poised to answer.

"I think I'm going to go on a date with Lloyd," I told our mutual friend Rob later in the Bowl.

"I don't think that's a good idea," Rob countered. "I wouldn't force it."

I knew what he was getting at. I'd just cut ties from a serious relationship, and I wasn't sure if I was attracted to Lloyd romantically. But didn't I deserve to know, to figure it out over sushi rolls or frozen custard? Wasn't it okay to say *yes* to a date as a pleasant curiosity? I didn't want to tame my curiosity. Behind me were too many serious, sad days.

It's hard to know your place in the world when azaleas thrive on acid, with soil pH somewhere between very strong and medium. I'd been living one pattern of love and relationship, and I needed to try a new way, a kinder way.

I left the library circulation desk to find a study spot. A couple hours later, Lloyd strolled by on official duty and paused beside me.

"Do you think anyone's ever spent the night in the library before?" I asked him. "I've always thought it would be fun to do before I graduate."

"How about Wednesday?" he said. The tips of my branches fluttered.

On Wednesday: we hide under a table in the microfilm room while the lights in the library are shut off one by one. There's the Rare Book Room, where Lloyd has stowed a sleeping bag and a backpack full of snacks, water, and flashlights. We sing "Circle of Life" musical theater style on the library's main stairwell, ascending. We plop down on '70s-brown carpet to read Dante's *Divina Commedia* aloud in Italian.

My roots clutch courage when I reach out to touch his neck with my fingertips. I run my fingers up and down those fine blond hairs and across the folds of his shoulder blades. He stays still, at my request. He closes his eyes and releases a downy exhale. I do not want to be watched or touched; I want only to dust his skin with my innocence and my freedom, do nothing with my tongue or my breasts or my thighs. To remember how it might feel to want to touch a person, to let fingers sweeten into new, safe clearings. His follicles swell up to meet the edges of my fingernails. Minutes breathe into more minutes, and my fingers spin slow ribbons. A flush of relief because he's receiving exactly what I want to give and not moving us toward anything *more*. I see his eyelids flickering like small wings in a chrysalis, and I know this is no small wonder for him too, something he needed to feel. One of us might cry before sunrise. We fall asleep in the deep quiet on the unzipped sleeping bag, as if cradled in the warm hollow of a tree, breath slow and full.

PLEASURE
TOLERANCE

I didn't need ghost stories as a child because I knew my
nana's body. In high school I interviewed her for a school
project, and I flew to Florida for the weekend to record her
story. Palm leaves swayed in the warm breeze while we sat
on her porch with tall glasses of milk splashed with Kahlúa.
The microcassette tape turned for eleven hours, and Nana
Jojo's words patched together unevenly, her French accent
stretching the syllables:

> *I had intestinal tuberculosis and I was full of tumors in my
> uterus. The doctor said, "It's you or the baby. Not both of you
> will make it." I said, "I choose my baby. I'm having this baby."
> They put me to sleep; I was asleep when she was born. People
> still thought she wouldn't make it when she came out. A priest
> came to anoint her with her last rites. She was all yellow, skin
> yellow, eyes yellow. What's it called?* Jaunisse. *They gave me a
> hysterectomy after birth; everything was too messed up from
> surgery and the TB and the tumors. They wouldn't let her
> drink my milk. They said it was no good because of the TB.*

The details lined up like stars as my nana talked, as if she remembered the story by looking up at the night sky and finding a constellation, flecks of light to make order of big darkness.

Of all her stories, I know this one the best:

In a hospital in Oran, Algeria, in 1954, my Nana Jojo, Simone Schmitt, is thirteen, and her abdomen gapes open. An appendectomy has gone wrong; her intestines were punctured. A nurse brings her a glass of sloshing red to drink in the morning. Horse blood. Next, the leeches, placed one by one on her open wound. Sucking, attaching. Another nurse fishes for worms in her belly. *Prepare an outfit for her; call a priest*, the doctor tells her mother, Marie.

Nine months she stays in the hospital bed with her belly an open wound. Her mother rides the bus to visit every day while her father gets drunk and smells like the perfume of other women. The Algerian War for independence begins while she lies there. First she hears the bombs, and then the clapping and shouting from the Arabic patients, segregated on the other side of the hospital.

"The nurses put—what's the word?—the thing from the mother and the baby." Her hands formed a circle in front of her the size of a cake.

"Placenta?"

"Yes, placenta." She shook her head and rolled her eyes for forgetting. "They put other people's placenta on the hole on my belly. Fresh placenta from the baby who had just been born."

My grandmother used the word *miracle* to describe it all: her survival, my mother's survival, the fact that I was able to be born at all.

By the time the interviews were over, I understood that if you want to believe in miracles, you must look straight into the grotesque eye of a wound until it is transfigured. The line between the horrific and the miraculous could be as thin as breath.

It's been two weeks since my last silver nitrate treatment, so I return for my third burning. I know now that when I leave, for days I will give off a metallic odor, like the taste of blood. I will feel my vagina turn to metal. Not cold, hard metal, but soft and molten.

As I pull up to the parking lot, I'm thinking about a story I heard on NPR recently. The piece interrogated the legacy of Dr. James Marion Sims, a nineteenth-century physician who has been called *the father of gynecology*. Sims invented the speculum and a surgical technique for the repair of a childbirth injury called a vesicovaginal fistula, a hole between the bladder and the vagina. Wondering if I had a fistula was why my own scars were discovered.

Although Sims was a trailblazer in a procedure that still helps women today, between 1846 and 1849 he performed experimental surgeries on enslaved women. Sims did not provide anesthesia for the ten Black women who were central to his research. Their pain was ignored, despite Sims's writing that Lucy, one of three women he names, "almost felt as if she were going to die, that she cried out in pain." After thirty surgeries on one woman, he finally succeeded in the technique.

I am alone in my car, one of the few times I've been alone this week, and in the silence I hear their names: *Anarcha. Lucy. Betsey.* The mothers of modern gynecology. The women whose bodies became living blazes in Sims's trail of discovery.

I wonder how soon after the surgeries the women had to return to the cotton fields or the household. I wonder how many hours they stood each day, if their organs felt like runny yolks between their legs, if their undergarments soaked through. I wonder if they were embarrassed of the smell, if people didn't want to eat beside them. I wonder if rashes gripped their thighs from the friction of sweat and urine. I wonder if what ripened under their dresses, yellow stains of heavy suns, protected them from rape.

No anesthesia is necessary for the silver nitrate treatments, but the words *discomfort* and *irritation* that Dr. S used on the first day are mild. Once Dr. S is in front of me with her rolling tray of silver nitrate, I ask for the mirror. This feels like courage, to admit that I still want more of this image. I could replay what I've seen twice before, but I need to see the long face of the truth again.

I watch a giant cotton probe move my inner folds to the side before a hand covers the scars with the silver. I hold the mirror like a woman who wants to speak to her ancestors, like a woman who wants to look upon all that has been neglected across centuries. To my great-grandmother who died in a labor camp in Cambodia after bearing two sons from the colonizer, sons recruited for French colonial wars when they came of age.

Tell the truth, body, vagina two generations removed from the colonizer. Lament and I will hold you. I will keep vigil for all the mothers who have felt soft claws at their vulva and whose pain remains invisible. What's invisible is relentless infinity. I do not accept this as our story. I hold the mirror like a woman who says, *Put your hand in mine and come.*

The next day I call my doula to ask her what she remembers about my second-degree tear. She says she watched my repair, and she didn't see anything unusual; it was very straightforward. The tissue seemed to line up well. She has worked at many births with my midwife and is sure that Lydia would never try to repair anything outside of her skill level; in fact, she's heard her tell some mothers she didn't feel comfortable performing a repair.

"I didn't expect to still have so much healing ahead of me at this point," I confess, sitting on my bed with the phone getting hot on my cheek during nap time. "It's a little confusing because emotionally, the birth left me feeling more peaceful and powerful. But physically the recovery has been so long and painful. I already had issues with my sexuality before this, and now I'm worried that sex will always be hard."

"It took a while for me to heal, too," she says. "This may sound strange, but even though the area was different after, I found I could experience even more pleasure."

I thank her and hang up the phone, sliding my fingers across the cheek smudge on the screen. From this cleft of hemorrhoids, incontinence, and burned scars, the word *pleasure* sounds like a distant slurry. Leaked on cotton panties, dried into human crust. As if it's running straight through me but it wants to stay.

A squirrel out the window chases another squirrel up a loblolly pine, and patches of bark drop down. I open Facebook and see a friend has posted an ultrasound photo with the caption: *Googles: How painful is childbirth?*

It's a pregnancy announcement. A laugh quakes from me. I also searched for answers to that question before giving birth, both the first time and the second since my first baby didn't come through my vagina. Today I feel a new question squeezing through, thrumming. I prepared for the pain of labor. I trained for birth like some train for triathlons. I summoned a team of four women wise to the energy of bursting water bags, thinning cervix, and stretching labia. They arrived with baskets full of comfort and safety measures, peanut balls for wedging my legs, rainbow-weave rebozos to sift my belly while I was on hands and knees, and sticks of amber honey to crack open and bead onto my tongue. I meditated several times a day for weeks until my cells seemed to whirr. I made a playlist of drumbeats for the mood of shaking baby down; I made a playlist of soothing chanteys; I made a playlist of empower-the-fuck-up queen bee anthems.

I welcomed pain onto my bedsheets, into my body, like a most honorable guest. Directly under the crown of dried flowers haloed with the white lace ribbons on the wall, my baby broke from me, like a Eucharist, I on my knees. My pain smelled like clary sage and was accompanied by a silky cloth blotting my cheeks with wetness. How beautiful my pain presented, how I courted it and shaped my body to frame its edges.

I can't question my pain tolerance. A 10.5-pound baby with a 99th percentile head carved through my vagina. I traveled to my limits of sensation and beyond in birth, a slither force rolling me out of myself. During transition, when I fully dilated, it felt as if my insides were being sucked out by a cosmic vacuum, while I spun in total loss of control. *I do not like this*, I told Lloyd when I found my voice. *I. do. not. like. this.*

With that same resilience at my center, a new invitation contracts the room.

You showed up for your pain. Will you show up for your pleasure too?

Without the birth moan, the great rock-heads of my babies splitting me, and the asphalt heat of the silver nitrate, pleasure would feel like a luxury. Nothing but a sugar cloud melting on my mouth. But today pleasure calls to me from my torn skin like a dare, like a sound I've never made.

Only because blood is snaking down its ankle do I believe pleasure's here for me.

I am nursing in bed, lying on my side, and my baby begins tapping his foot like a metronome against my thigh. *Tap Tap Tap.* A reverberation travels inward, slipping into the V of my legs. A little tingle travels up my front and curls in me like warmth. *Do I stop his foot from tapping? Am I a pedophile if this feels good?* I wonder. *Does the pleasant feeling have to be bad?*

Veronica told me to do my Kegels while sitting, driving, nursing. I can feel my muscles getting stronger, and just doing a few deep vagina squeezes can slide a ripple up my spine now.

I never have an urge to touch my baby inappropriately or to act on the sensations in a sexual way. All I do is imagine my vagina as a tissued hand lifting a blueberry. Or as an elevator traveling slowly up to the top floor and then back down to the ground floor. All I do is close my eyes and write poetry about the fruit stem plucking deep inside me. *My vagina is a ripe tomato pulling on the vine. It is the thin skin of a chrysalis when the butterfly starts to stretch its wings.*

orb-weaver spider

A tattoo is a wound we give ourselves. We adorn ourselves with the wound. Sophia and I drove to the tattoo shop by the railroad tracks downtown. I had two words emblazoned across the left side of my ribs: *VITA NOVA*. A swallow flew straight into the letters. Sophia got the same words on her wrist, in the script of our favorite poetry collection by Louise Glück, tender lines we often read aloud to each other. As the needle punctured my skin, I lay sweating on the table, eyes wide open.

"Wow, you're handling this well," Erica the tattoo artist told me. "The ribs are one of the most painful spots."

This was pain I could choose. This was the pain of new life. But more than pain I could choose, it was myself I chose, my own skin that I flew toward, singing *New new new*. After, I looked at my flesh in the mirror, with the strong, serifed letters and the beak pointing forward, and saw something I chose.

I chose more than needles to caress me. I was in love. From a hollowed-out tree, honey opened from me, learning

Lloyd, and Lloyd learning me. Love felt soon, but the soon felt palm-open, not fist-closed soon. The word *rebound* bit me every now and then, but I kissed its teeth, knowing it didn't match the rhythm of my heart. My greatest wonder: that I could trust my heart, not a flimsy filament, but a wise, sturdy pump that knew how to convert blood oxygen-poor to blood oxygen-rich.

A few days after the tattoo, I sat wearing my cap and gown in the full Mississippi sun in the Bowl while waiting to walk across the stage. Under my black gown was the raw, inked flesh blotting my ribs, covered with plastic wrap and streaked with bloody sweat. The itch skimmed my skin like ant legs.

There were things I knew that J had taken from me, shadows the bright sun forced across the grass. Across the rows of graduates, I smiled at people who never became as close as I thought they would after my life bisected. My honors project about French-Algerian women writers had become unmanageable, so I wore no honorary hood.

I sweated into my polyester regalia in the Bowl, the sun mudding the caves of my armpits, but I focused my attention on the itchy whirr of the swallow's wings against my rib bones. What I didn't choose felt small and shrunken next to all the choices still ahead of me.

My home for the summer was my grandmother Addie's old house in the suburbs, which had a faint end-of-life smell. The Summertree House was fully furnished with a forest-green formal dining room, a juicer, and decades of faded tea towels and recipe clippings. Neighbors mowed and hedged, kids clapped yard-play sounds, and middle-aged speed-walkers rounded the cul-de-sac. I had three bedrooms, so Sophia

and our friend Bernadette moved in too, along with a taran-
tula Bernadette had caught on a biology field mission in the
Arizona desert.

I hadn't spent the night at the Summertree House since
my grandma died the year before, months when I drove her
to radiation and chemo, when I learned to flush her saline IV
port and to empty her living-room commode. Before she got
really sick, I once saw her dancing alone in her living room
before I rang the doorbell. The lively rhythm of salsa per-
cussed through the glass. My grandma's house was one of
the few places I could go without J's protest. When I wasn't
in class or working on the newspaper, I was always caring for
someone: my preschool students, my grandma, J.

But this summer was my time.

"Has his life been hard enough for him to really *get* you?"
Sophia asked as we wove around the neighborhood. We
liked to walk the one-mile loop in the evening. I pondered
her question. Lloyd's childhood had been happy, with strong
and fond family relationships and no major trauma. I'd seen
a card that his father tenderly signed *Dad(dy)* and knew that
he had a tradition of running his hometown's Gum Tree 10K
with his mother. With his sisters, there were favorite songs
shared on mixed CDs and toothy smiles as he described their
personalities.

Since I was a little girl, I'd bonded with friends and family
over sorrow. The way to get close to a person was to know
how the world had broken their heart, the ache that carved
them into being. It was the way I'd bonded with J and with
many friends too. As freshmen, Sophia and I had bonded over
music, films, journalism, and poetry, but we'd also bonded
over processing the sorrows and transgressions of our child-
hoods in daring ways that felt newly possible once we moved

out of our family homes and into the dorms. I could see what Sophia was asking: Did Lloyd have the emotional patina to appreciate and connect with me? Could we bond on a deep level if our histories were so different? A *hard enough life* signified a finely textured emotional fabric threaded by a history of struggle, and the question was: could our textures work together, each one of us fully seen and appreciated?

I thought back to what I learned after our first kiss. Lloyd had walked me back to my dorm from the library. He leaned in, and I leaned in. But the moment his lips met mine, my chest went stony. My tongue grew too big in my mouth. I felt my body slip away from me and into J's control, and immediately I felt nauseous, as if J could see me. His voice grew mold spores in my head: *You're a little slut, aren't you?*

The kiss was brief, and I said *Good night*, slipping a smile from my mouth as I swiped my card at the door.

The next day, I walked over to Lloyd's dorm and knocked on his door.

"I need to talk to you. Can we go somewhere?" He followed me across the parking lot, where I stopped next to a construction zone, the grating of metal behind us. My fingers grasped the chain-link fence as I spoke.

"I know I told you you could kiss me, but I'm actually not ready to be physical with anyone. I thought I was ready, but I'm not." He knew I had recently ended a long-term relationship. I vowed to do everything differently—no secrets, no withheld feelings, and no ambivalent physical intimacy. I searched for disappointment or frustration in Lloyd's eyes, but I didn't see it.

"Take as long as you need. I'll follow your lead," he said.

"It's just . . . I went through a lot in my last relationship. It didn't end well. I'm sorry to be so complicated." My voice listed, the question in me stumbling: *Who's going to want someone as broken as me?* An excavator moved shelves of orange dirt from one pile to another. He didn't look away. "Catherine, I don't have a rubric in my head of what I want you to be. This is not an à la carte situation—take this part of you, leave the rest. I want to know all of you. I'm happy to just be able to spend time with you, whatever that looks like." His blue eyes bloomed in the distance between us. I wondered if he could hear the birdsong through my body. Could he feel my roots spreading wide like fingers, my trunk relaxing into steady fullness? I wondered if he could hear generations of men laying down their weapons in beds of pine to look skyward and say, *How beautiful.*

I held this memory in mind next to Sophia's question as we walked. My feet swished on the pavement.

"I don't know if his life has to be hard for him to get me," I told her. "I think he does get me. I mean, J's life was pretty hard, and did he get me?"

Maybe my suffering wasn't what made me most essentially me, I was also beginning to see. When I'd left J in February, I felt compacted into the worst person I had ever been. Dishonest, secretive, alienated, incapable of loving someone in a way that actually made him feel loved. I was cold, hard-packed earth. Now I felt close to the silty river loam, rich home for a fig tree ready to fruit. A warm core of joy and trustworthiness rose up my spine.

But the peace I felt didn't survive the night. I worried, turning from my left side to my right in my grandparents' old California king bed, tufted with faded pink velvet on the headboard. The years of abuse felt like a contagion within me that would infect Lloyd, catch fever between us. I worried his parents wouldn't like me if they knew my history, as if I were warbling the protractor-straight arc of their only son's Eagle Scout life. I felt like a newly sober addict in recovery, well intentioned but unpredictable, with the inertia in me written toward toxicity, a chemical dependency on dysfunction. I'd watched the vector of pain in my parents' relationship and in those of the women I loved. Lloyd never had a thirty-five-year-old step-grandfather who pointed a finger and spattered, *Fuck you*, while he packed boxes to help his grandmother leave him. Lloyd's dad had never asked him to stay home from school to keep his mother company so she wouldn't take too many pills. I located myself within these whiffs of danger.

I had watched the dysfunction reproduce between J and me, as if my heart were worm-bloated and destined to fail. If I hadn't been able to stop it then, what might sneak through now? As the sheet twisted around my legs, sweat wrapped me, and I was the swamp—slippery water moccasin, disease-carrying mosquito—next to Lloyd's freshwater stream. It's only the female mosquitoes who drink our blood, I learned, needing the feast to produce their eggs. Male mosquitoes don't even have mouthparts strong enough to pierce animal skin.

Was I needy and desperate, feeding off Lloyd's health, attaching myself to his vitality and innocence? He was a virgin. He'd never had a girlfriend before. I felt as if I'd already been privately married and drained by twenty-one, as if I'd become a Walking Wounded Widow. I had adopted a shelter dog with J, and my name was on the internet service account. Maybe someone healthier wouldn't allow herself to fall in love only three months after leaving an abusive relationship. Maybe she would declare independence and embark on a solo backpacking trip across Europe. I wasn't supposed to already be imagining what it would be like to be part of his family, playing Bananagrams. Maybe this was not a thing that responsible people allowed themselves to feel.

Next the Femme Fatale rushed into my grandparents' cream-scrolled bed with me. Maybe I was the reviled woman who ensnares men with her eroticism and doesn't let them go. Seductress. Predator. The Sirens could veer Odysseus's sailors off their course and lure them to the rocks, making them lose all notion of self and home. What about that surprise blow job in the car before graduation? It fell well within the purview of sexy new relationship energy, but did I really want it or was I only luring Lloyd closer, casting a spell over him? Did I want *him* or did I want the power? The orb-weaver spider makes a zigzag pattern across her web to attract prey. Enchantress. Man Eater.

Maybe I wasn't that different from J. That's what I feared in my swampiest moments.

My heartbeat chased worry in my chest, great long legs running. Suddenly the fears twisted in me, and I was the one being eaten. A door in the bedroom with a panel of sheer glass led to the backyard patio. The backyard's darkness could be hiding a face. J knew the Summertree House; he'd been here for Christmas when my grandma was alive. If he drove by, he'd see my Honda Element in the driveway. The old mattress creaked under me as I strained against the chase in my head, imagining I was being watched. I turned my face away from the door, but still I imagined the glass shattering, the door breached by a man who thought he had a right to me. *This is very unlikely. This is not in touch with reality. He would never do that*, I thought. The coil of a metal spring pushed against my thigh. I remembered other things I never thought he would do, and the known world and its laws of gravity trembled.

Lloyd invited me to visit him at the summer camp where he was working as a nature guide. He wrote skits, led trail hikes, sang songs, ran in chase games, and spun ghost stories. Even though it was less than an hour away from the Summertree House, he was in a whole different world, might as well have been The Big Rock Candy Mountains, with ice cream scoop clouds and lemon squeeze sun. I knew he felt connected to his truest self here, and I wanted to see him in his element.

When I arrived at lunchtime, there was a buzz of *Lloyd's girlfriend* in the humid air. I didn't mind the word *girl-friend* now, even though when Lloyd first floated it, the word squeezed my neck like a choke collar because I'd been a girlfriend only once, and it almost killed me. "How about Adventure Duo?" I suggested with a smile, and for weeks we rolled like river otters in this definition of our own making, until it became clear that the word *girlfriend* could also have a definition of our own making, built new by us.

When I pulled up, he was waiting for me in the parking lot in a neon-yellow T-shirt, khaki shorts, and Tevas. On his shirt: a heart wrapped in duct tape that said, *Stick it together with the tape, the tape of love.* His smile was free and easy, waiting for me in the June sun. He wrapped me in a hug, and I remembered the honey goodness of us, the way he made me want to stick my hands in the dirt and make something live. The way a stranger at McDade's Market had stopped us in the cereal aisle to say, *Y'all look like you could change the world together*, and I declared, *We can.*

I'd missed him, but I knew the distance was good for us. It was the kind of distance I'd wanted to have with J, for us to take our own separate adventures and return more ourselves. Lloyd lived in a house full of ten girls and ecstatic camp theatrics, and whenever I felt left behind, I willed myself to remember Greece and France, how much I had needed the freedom. I had the chance to be the person I wanted to be now, the girlfriend who would freely give Lloyd the space to do what he loved. So I let the clenched feelings sweat out of me at home, and when I missed him, I wrote letters that arrived in envelopes that I collaged with '60s-era *National Geographic* magazines. Still, it felt like getting clean. Like withdrawal. Painful.

We stepped into the dining hall for sloppy joes. After, we sang songs and stomped, a counselor got a bucket of ice water dumped on his head, and then the staff jumped onto the tables to announce the afternoon's activities. Lloyd jumped into the center ring.

"Heeeey, everybody!" he called, swinging his arm through the air.

"Heeeey, Lloyd!" everybody called back in singsong unison.

"Today in Nature marks the CULMINATION of a dangerous journey to TASTY rewards," he announced. "We have DUG the mud from the STICKIEST edges of the camp woods, and SLATHERED it, layer by layer, to make our mud oven. Now, come join us as we bring FIRE to light this oven and stoke the hot coals. 'Cause tonight it's time to BAKE BLACKBERRY PIE!!"

I followed him to the oven, where we gathered sticks and leaves for the fire. Lloyd crouched with his cheek almost touching the earth to blow breath into the sparks. As the fire got hotter, we watched the mud on the outside transform from a dark, seedy brown to a sandy color, seeping smoke. The oven worked.

"Time to get blackberries," he told me after the kids ran to their cabins for rest period. "Wanna ride with me in the truck?" His eyebrows arched, and he motioned toward an old, green pickup truck parked by the riding lawnmower and the utility barn.

"Umm, yeah. Of course." I was overwhelmed by a sense of belonging. I was here, right here, with him and with Mississippi's fruits. I became aware of dreams for us, some as small as a blackberry and some as big as forever. Even in the beginning, my mind and heart had never allowed me to imagine being with J forever even when I tried; an ending always loomed over us. This *forever* dream was new. Along with the feeling that loving Lloyd made me want to be the best person I could be, and I believed I could actually be her.

We hopped in, and he drove us across the main road to the extended camp property. I scooted close to him on the bench seat, and he wrapped his arm around my shoulder.

"I've never driven a lady in a truck before," he said, cracking a smile.

"I can't say I've had the pleasure either." I hammed up the Southern charm.

He took us off-road and down a widely mowed trail. He knew exactly where to find the blackberries; he ran these trails. Once we were down the hill and out of view, I leaned in for a kiss, our mouths salty from summer and smoky from the oven's fire. I lay my head on his shoulder near the muddy musk of his armpit.

"Now, the three threats of blackberry picking are fire ants, poison ivy, and briar thorns," he cautioned before we got out. "The fruit doesn't come without risk."

"Got it. I'm not afraid," I flashed back.

"Oh—and wasps. That's the fourth."

By the time we got back in the truck, his nose was bright red and my shoulder was too, so I knew that sunburn was the fifth. But our cut-off plastic milk jugs were full of summer's good flesh, and I slipped one purple-stained finger in my mouth, sucking on the skin a thorn had opened.

I found the growth while I was in the shower, in the summer month when the magnolia petals turn brown. It was a rubbery roundness in my breast that I could move with the pad of my finger. Within a few days, surgery was scheduled to remove the mass and determine if it was a threat.

"We'll figure this out," Lloyd said over the phone from camp. "I mean, *you'll* figure it out."

"I liked the *we*," I said.

My mom flew to town and would tend to me on the day of my surgery. Knowing she would see my naked torso after surgery, I told her about my tattoo. I lifted my shirt.

"Why'd you have to get something so big?" she gasped, her head rearing back like a threatened snake. She had a tattoo on the small of her back, but it was one small letter: X. Mine wrapped around my side like a panel of armor or a folded wing. She looked stunned, horrified. She wandered to the kitchen and started opening the cabinets. She came back to the bedroom with a half-empty bottle of tequila, nursing it all evening while her mascara ran from her eyelashes.

I'd recently told her the truth of what happened with J. We sat in a snack house on campus called Reuben's, where I found a spot for us, alone in the back room. I looked to the side as I spoke, the intensity of her eye contact crushing, but every now and then I caught a glimpse of her face. Her eyebrows furrowed like the Madonna in paintings of her seven sorrows.

Even as she reached out to hug me, saying, "Why didn't you tell me?," I wanted to be strong for her. She held on tightly, tears making wet stars of her eyes, and I wanted to assure her, *Mom, I wouldn't let anyone save me. Remember? You tried to tell me to break up with him when we sat in the parking lot at Walmart when I came to visit in California. And I wouldn't hear it. I got mad. I refused to talk about it.*

After I showed her the tattoo, I could see she was grieving something more than the ink on my skin. She'd held my seven-pound-fourteen-ounce body as a newborn and named me Catherine after herself. Things had happened to my body since then, scary things she couldn't protect me from even though she had raised me in the school of fierce daughters.

In surgery the next day, my mom and dad waited together outside the operating room, brought together by the invasive mass in my body. Since Dad was a pathologist at this hospital, immediately after the mass was excised from my breast, my parents walked to the lab. They watched the surgical pathologist, who lunched regularly with my dad, slice into the mass, scrape tissue for slides, and observe the cells under the microscope. Dad and his friend might have described what they saw like this: *abundant spindle stromal cells and naked nuclei, epithelium arranged in antler horn clusters.*

My mother's description: *It was very big, like a golf ball. It was black like coal.*

It was benign. It was out of me. But it made sense that something monstrous had grown in my body while I was with J. By the time I woke up in recovery, my parents were calm and smiling over my bed. "Hi, sweetie," my mom said as she stroked my hair.

THE SKIN BRIDGE

I ask Dr. S if we can bring out the mirror to look at my tear area together before my fourth silver nitrate treatment. If I'm going to have my vagina burned, at least I can use this time to learn about my body's changes.

I point to a stretch of skin that runs across the base of my vagina. "I've been wondering if this was there before or if this came from where I tore," I say. When I pull my butt cheek, the skin stretches up like a dam that I don't recall feeling before birth.

"That's from the repair," Dr. S says, explaining that extra skin was pulled into the stitching of my perineum. *A skin bridge*, she calls it.

"That explains why it feels so tight." I nod in a revelation that feels adjacent to wonder, my body becoming articulate. "It feels like I have a corset cinched there."

"That's exactly what it looks like," she says, her voice bright and affirming. "With time and intercourse, it will loosen up and stretch more."

"What's this?" I ask next. I direct her to nether holes above the skin bridge. She says those are a couple divots from the repair. "Are they closed?" I ask.

"I don't know. Let's check." She asks if she can put one gloved finger in my anus. From the outside, she dips the wooden end of the Q-tip into the slump to check its depth and terminus. Now I understand why I've been confused by the two pockets of skin that I've called *fool's butthole* and why, as I'm potty training Guider, I'm also learning how to wipe my butt again to avoid the bridge's pockets and the buttonholes. My underwear has become an embarrassment of stains, and many times I think that I've wiped thoroughly only to find surprise odors and slickness an hour later.

I still find it hard to believe that we don't talk more about the ways our bodies change after birth. Out beyond the standard, polite fare of stretch marks and baby weight, many of us have entirely new genital constructions and organs of waste that bulge into our vaginas.

Mommy body love has become a social media movement, where drooping belly folds and steri-taped C-section scars receive applause emojis and thousands of shares. We're opening our hearts to the mother wound, to rust lines of blood. But even in the midst of this stadium-sized wave of body acceptance, I linger horrified in the bathroom. It's not standing in front of the mirror and *liking what I see* that is The Journey. That feels like a sensible course, one that I've practiced since I was a prepubescent girl with an ear-length bob and a belly that pudged against my sunflower dress. It's not as a spectator that I struggle with my body. It's as an exiled inhabitant, a newcomer feeling like *a stranger in a strange land.*

Shame slips hallway notes into my palm with messages like *You're gross* and *You're broken beyond repair* and *Don't let your mother-in-law wash your undies—what will she think?* But I won't keep shame's secrets. I need to let them out before they make echoes in me.

"The skin bridge!" Morgan exclaims on the phone as I sit in the purple chair in the nursery. "Oh my god! The skin bridge! My friend Vera had this after her birth."

"Wait, you know about the skin bridge? This is a thing? Vera had it?" I stand up from my chair and walk between the changing table and the window. I immediately feel like less of a freak. Vera has a high-powered director job and is a vibrant woman who lowers into a full squat to throw her arms open wide to greet her toddler at daycare. Just knowing that Vera is living her life with a skin bridge in her pants makes me feel less like a mutant. She birthed her baby in a hospital, so I also know this could have happened no matter where I birthed, no matter who repaired me.

As Morgan talks, my right foot rubs the shaggy white carpet in the nursery, my toes smoothing the tangled clumps that have become gray with constant foot travel in the last three years of motherhood. Two worn, packed trails diverge at the corner of the rug from the door: one to the changing table and one to the purple nursing glider. The compacted shag tells a story of the care of bodies—other bodies.

She tells me about her recovery from her tear that striated up to her clitoris and how she was afraid of penetrative sex for more than a year. "When I was six months postpartum and still in so much pain, my doctor looked me in the eye, took my hand, and said, 'Morgan, this is common but it is not normal. You do not need to live with this pain. You do not have to accept this pain like so many women do.'"

When I move certain ways, sharpness still pinches me like a rat trap at my vulva. Other times, a sudden tug at the tightest spot of the repair halts me as if I've snagged on a serrated edge of a saw.

As Morgan and I talk and even laugh about the scars of our bodies, we give ourselves the name *vag-angelists*. I feel us actively breaking a cycle of wounding. The silence. When Morgan and I first met at a community mother blessing event, we were both pregnant with our first babies. She would later tell me that, in a room full of white women, she was immediately drawn to me as someone "racially ambiguous" or "ambiguously Brown" like she was. She was closely connected to her Puerto Rican and mixed heritage, and to hear her name her early perception of me as a mixed woman—and her sense of belonging in my presence—made me feel like part of a mixed community in a way I had never felt before. It feels right that now we're also coming into an open and shared understanding together of our private bodily changes in motherhood.

In nature, moss drinks up rainfall, absorbs toxins, and cleanses the soil in a way that allows the other plants around it to thrive. It's why my artist friend Sarah Jené collaborated on a grief-focused art installation called *Moss Couch*, a living repose made of moss and flowers patchworked over a reclaimed couch.

The artist note says: *Like grief, moss is persistent. It also plays a vital role in the development of new ecosystems.*

When I get off the phone, I feel as if the moss couch has embraced me. Birth changes bodies. Motherhood leaves its tendrils in our flesh, creating a new ecosystem. Maybe my body is healing messily not because something went wrong but because this is the order of bodies. Creation and destruction are clasped hands within the same circulatory system. When we're in it alone, our minds can tell us that our healing is messier than the healing of those around us. But our bodies are not machines, predictable, uniform, and following directions. Our bodies are wild, defiant, and willful. They keep on absorbing. They keep on remaking.

I am lying in bed while the kids are napping. I start tapping my thigh to see if I can produce the shimmery shiver I've felt from the baby's tapping foot. I can. I tap, and the vibration uncoils into my center. I move closer to my pelvis, tapping with the pad of my finger as if circling the rim of a singing bowl. I'm not looking for an orgasm; I just finger walk the mound of my sex to remember that feeling good is an option in my body. Through my underwear, I trace the outline of my labia. I press down with my middle finger, and each spot gets fluttery. The lower part where I tore is still painful to touch, radiating from the flaming pearl.

After my first birth, another mother described the year after her C-section as the sensation of *walking around as a floating head.* I even posted in a local moms' Facebook group about this feeling: a deadness in my womb space, a total lack of vitality between my belly button and my genitals. Today the area from my belly button down shimmers with sensation, alive.

For months the pain has called my attention. But alongside the pain shivers delight. It's not just the baby's tapping foot while he nurses. The other day I was dancing to music in the kitchen, and my backside grazed the edge of the counter. A vibration like a sunshaft pulsed into my clitoris. It's as if my birth tear has laid a band of new sensation from my anus, up my vulva, to my clitoris—some kind of *kintsugi* of the flesh, a golden seam over the tissue my baby tore through. The skin bridge.

I hear Hemingway's line that *The world breaks every one and afterward many are strong at the broken places.* I hear Leonard Cohen singing about how light slips through every crack. I've often wanted to push back on these lines, to assert that I also feel shakier at the broken places, that the broken places have accumulated handfuls of ER bills that have gone to collections. And other things have scurried through the cracks that have not been light. Cockroaches with big wings and long antennas, arriving hungry. Threads of smoke that swirl images, doubts, sensations.

When I try to grasp at answers, to solve for x and balance what's been lost with what's been found, the solutions slip through the crack too. My sentences trail off and end in echoes of who I was and who I thought I would be, what I love about myself and how complex trauma restructured my brain in ways that still hurt me and my family.

But what I have today is my body, my hand on my pelvis. I don't know what to do other than to stay close to it, finding what I find and making the life I can from the tangle of findings. When I quiet the voices of Hemingway and Cohen so I don't need to argue with them, I hear the voice of my body. My genitals are telling me, through sensation, that pleasure doesn't have to happen in the absence of pain. They can exist at the same time, in the same nerve endings. My scars, markers of history, are also actively shaping what's possible.

Pleasure felt artificial and saccharine before this pain, like too-sweet taffy stuck to my molars, pretty in its colorful package but less than tasty in my mouth. The substance of pleasure is changing, though, becoming sustenance.

Pleasure is a week's wages brought home as food. Pleasure is coming with the force of my great-grandma Rosalina, an Italian immigrant who lost her husband in a coal mine and was left with six kids. She's washing the laundry for her family by hand and ironing every piece of it, even underwear and sheets. Pleasure's coming with the resilience of my great-grandmother Marie giving birth to her fifth daughter while her husband came home smelling like perfume and grunting, *Another girl?*, without even asking to see her newborn face. Pleasure is coming from the women whose blood made me, with that same devotion. I want to fight for every shred of the pleasure we deserve.

There was a moment when Dr. S asked me about birth control, and I realized that a part of me was wondering if she was disgusted at the prospect that my husband—any man—could find me desirable in this state. How could this gross body even participate in sexuality? But pleasure isn't coming for me now with the force of Photoshop strangers behind it, a spectacle curated for others to admire, the production of what other people want to see of me through a hole in the wall. Pleasure isn't the sister of *pleasing*. Pleasure is heaving up from this mother body. With sharp and yeasty nipples that burn as if glazed with ground glass. With a vagina that can't be entered because scars are falling from it with a sizzle.

Pleasure comes saying, *All* that *and still* this. *This is yours. You belong here.*

No one ever tells you: Masturbate while the baby sleeps. Conventional wisdom says, *Sleep*. But in the middle of winter, my body begins to hum with desire. A beehive lives inside my pelvis, and a constant buzz of pleasure pursues me through my day. The more I notice it, the more I look for it, and the more often it finds me. At a stoplight, the low rumbling vibration of the car makes a tightness at my center where the seam of my jeans holds me.

In my last pelvic PT session, Veronica used a vaginal sensor and loaded an image of a blooming rose on the computer screen. As I contracted my muscles and released, I could watch the rose respond. As I squeezed, the petals closed inward, as if returning to a bud. When I released, the rose opened, full and velvety.

Before long, I lie in bed and rub my labia until my orgasm crests in ripples of eight, nine, ten waves. I've never felt such layered and exquisite orgasms. For the first time, I notice the contractions of an orgasm. I feel the way the muscles flare—open and close, open and close—like the rose opening and closing in fast motion. A whole palette of orgasms begins to appear to me: orgasms that are long and short, pulsing and intense, quiet flashes and flickers. Rather than rating one kind as better than the others, I begin to appreciate the multiplicity.

One day I discover that the flat pressure of my palm on the mound of my old C-section scar feels like velvet bunching attached to my clitoris. I move the heel of my hand in gentle circles on the mound, and the velvet gathers between my legs. Is the webbing of scar tissue from my old C-section pulling on my clitoris? I've had this scar for more than two years, but I've never felt something alive here, rings of velvet blooming.

"Your body is exciting and new," Lloyd has told me. He's been giving me the look a lot recently, the look as if he can't wait for consent to palm every inch. The look tells me I'm luscious. The look tells me I'm round in new ways and curving with breasts like a fertility goddess. The look tells me that we went from having sex multiple times in twenty-four hours to try to get labor started to having almost no sex for six months.

But my body's ache is not for another body; my body's ache is for my own. And since my scars' chemical flames would burn my partner's penis, for the first time, I let myself want only myself, warm and moving.

snowflakes

When the snow arrived, sleep was over. A knock at my door. Lloyd's dancing eyes, irises packed crystal blue. It was easy to say *yes* to the snow dragon, to building it together, to rushing into the swath of flakes that swirled. We're not prepared for snow like this in Mississippi, so I bundled up in what I had. Over the layers, I threw my red rain cape with the hood that made me feel as if I were traveling through the dark wood to grandmother's house. But I was not entering the dark wood; I'd come through it.

February again. One year since I escaped, almost exactly.

I was living on campus as a college employee, granted an apartment and meal points, which meant I often texted Lloyd before midnight to say *Hungry?* and ten minutes later he'd meet me at Reuben's for a chicken quesadilla. It felt like a bonus year of college, makeup for the time I'd missed in my off-campus life with J.

Lloyd and I crunched through snow ankle-deep to reach the untouched field for our snow dragon, out past the snow highways trampled by sorority Uggs and the iced-over sidewalks lined with five-minute, quickie snowmen. When we rolled the first snowballs, we didn't know the creature's whole architecture, but we knew we were building something big. That's how we were. Not settling for expected forms but imagining fantastical possibilities.

Dragons were more Lloyd's thing than mine. He had a bumper sticker on his PT Cruiser that said, *Do not meddle in the affairs of dragons, for you are crunchy and good with ketchup.* But I appreciated the paradox of form and content: ice crystals, the dragon's fire. Lloyd began with the chest piece, a big scoop of snow that he rolled into a stately mass. I packed bulk until its shoulders were almost as high as ours.

Over the summer, at a lake house after our friends went to bed, I'd told Lloyd the violence that J did to me. The winter night of the pepper spray, a hand gripping my wrist, my mouth cracked open. Lloyd didn't look away as my voice shook. I asked him if it was too hard to hear the graphic details. He said it was hard but that he would listen to whatever I wanted him to know. His eyes formed full, round tears as I spoke. When they slipped down his cheeks, he didn't brush them off; they shone, my witnesses. His tears didn't ask for my comfort either. He held me, and I felt held. It felt less as if he was seeing a wound exposed and more as if he was seeing me. Maybe that's when I knew: *What is ahead of me will be very different from what is behind me.*

Once we shaped the bust, with dragon shoulders erect like a sphinx, we walked behind it to map the scale of body and tail. Lloyd used the edge of his hiking boot to trace a rough outline on the ground.

"Yeah? What do you think?" He motioned with his arm to a tail that would end more than twenty feet from the head. With a couple studio art classes on his transcript, he had a good handle on perspective and proportion.

"Let's do it," I nodded, tipping my eyebrows to accept his proposal. I didn't feel as if I took a supporting role to his idea; this was our project. I did admire his confidence, though, the quick draw of speaking his ideas, a product of being male and raised in a household where dissenting opinions on theology were encouraged, along with the familial ease of reciting favorite *Seinfeld* scenes. I wanted to watch his confidence and learn from it, not like gold foil that would rub off on me but like a palette we would share, dipping my brush into shades he knew to blend, that our culture had encouraged him to blend.

I knew it would take hours to build a snow creature of this scale, but the snow fell like a pleasure all around us, and we would figure out the structure together.

It wasn't just J in my dark woods. It was a pattern of older men and the heightened intensity of secret romance. Even before I met J, I wrote a little ditty of a poem in my journal that wandered down the page like party confetti.

> Catherine, why
> is
>   it
> that   every
>   time
> you l ook
>   for a
>   boy   friend
> you find
>   a man
>   friend
> in stead?

My first kiss was with a nineteen-year-old French bohe-
mian named Gaëtan, whose face launched a thousand reggae
songs. I was fourteen going on fifteen, traveling to France
for a family wedding, and we met in the pews of a Picardie
cathedral. We didn't speak the same language, not fluently,
but our eyes did. Our hands did when his fingers found mine,
sticky from beurre and Brie. He guided me to the backyard In
the middle of a family party, where I was staying in the hills
above Paris, and by the blackberry bushes at the peach-nec-
tar of golden hour, he kissed me. *First French kiss, here with
a French boy,* I thought. *Perfect.* His tongue was pierced with
a silver knot like a tied cherry stem, and he was shirtless,
vagabond tan, with a blade-edged tattoo under the hairs by
his belly button. His face looked initiated, as if he had seen
the light. My fingers swelled in the summer heat, and in the
bathroom after, I struggled to get a ring over my knuckle
that I wanted off once I knew it was stuck. Gaëtan slipped
my finger into his mouth and ran his tongue along the edges
of metal, eyes meeting mine. From my lips he drew no sound,
but from my center he drew wanting.

After I returned home, I composed emails for months
with my hardbound French–English dictionary at my side.
Gaëtan was the real reason I learned to speak French, not
my lineage, not my mother, not Mireille with her *Mystères et
boule de gomme* in my school's Language Lab videos. But he
was too busy being free in the French countryside, sleeping in
his camion and plucking wine grapes from heirloom vines on
the *vendange.* I was left with the stretchy black headband he
gave me, which held the large safety pin he cocked like a bar-
rette and the old-book smell of his curls. Sometimes I slept
with his headband on my pillow, sliding the safety pin back

and forth. I imagined what might happen in his camion if I ever had the chance again.

A couple years later, there was Mark, twenty-nine and a Black Rastafarian. We met at an African dance class. He played djembe, and I raised my arms to the heavens to praise the sun, shook them toward the floor to sow seeds. When I danced, I saw him watching me in the mirror. Sometimes our eyes met in the glass face of our reflections. After the first class, I started wearing mini biker shorts to practice. *Ride the horse*, the teacher called, *ride the horse*, and I rocked my hips as if I knew what I was doing, following the jubilant gallop of the drums. Mark and I began chatting on the phone; one night he asked me, *Are you sure you're white? You don't have the soul of a white woman.* His voice felt so low it must have been stitched into the grass. It made my skin tingle.

Mark invited me to a local charity festival to watch him play drums. They had a bounce house and cotton candy. Puppies were available for adoption.

Have you ever touched a penis? No.

Even better—

Have you ever seen a penis? I hadn't.

He liked this. He knew he had quite a specimen to show me after we burned to the end of the blunt. I felt like a first-time pianist being invited to play on a Steinway grand. I held it in my hand and knew it was massive, something I should like, but I felt no pleasure stir in me.

That's when Mom found me in the back of Mark's white van in the parking lot of the coffee shop where I'd told her I was going. I wore the brown spaghetti-strap shirt without a bra she'd told me not to wear. Minutes later, Dad was at my mom's door, as if she'd called an ambulance.

Did he touch you? Dad asked. *You can tell me if he touched you.* I summoned steadiness in my pupils. *No,* I said. Soon I heard Dad's voice on the phone with Mark as I sat in the kitchen: *Stay away from my daughter. She's sixteen.* He sounded eerily calm, like someone removing a bomb with surgical precision.

I still talked with Mark for months. I'd sneak out of girl-choir practice every Monday and call him on the landline at the desk in the church lobby. I mailed him long letters that I dropped in post office boxes with no return address.

Later when J and I talked about this, I told him, "I think Mark happened so that I would learn how to better hide our relationship."

"That's what I was thinking," he said. "It was destiny."

I'd been such a careful little girl. I kept the stickers intact on my Beatrix Potter sticker sheet because I didn't want to paste the sticker on a spot I'd later regret. I moved from being that little girl to a teenager whose dad said, "It's a slippery slope, Catherine, a slippery slope." A drug test chilled perpetually in our fridge, and though he never asked me to pee in the cup, it remained next to the milk carton like a sentry. "I'd hate for something to happen to you," he said.

Something. Something had happened.

I didn't want to be the careful little girl who was afraid to use her stickers nor did I want to be the teenager who snuck around with forbidden men. I wanted to build something beautiful and shameless in the bright light of day.

The snow was beginning to melt through my gloves and burn my fingers as we built the dragon, but it didn't keep Lloyd and me from singing about making little birdhouses in our souls. Even the burning wetness of my fingers felt like a spark, a call to shine. Before I reached down to scoop a ball for the dragon's tail, I turned the ring on my finger so the yellow sapphire wouldn't pinch my skin under my glove. Emerald cut, flanked by baguette diamonds in my grand-mother's platinum setting. Lloyd had talked with my father, obtained my grandma's ring from the family safe, took it to the jeweler, and picked out a new gem.

He had proposed before the new year, reading me an original poem called "Prisms" in front of a hundred high schoolers at Winter Solstice camp. When he got down on one knee, the room became a decadent soar of pubescent screams. It was easy to say *yes*. Only a few months into dating when I had first visited his childhood home, we cuddled on the couch, and I told him, *I want to talk to you for the rest of my life.* What this also meant: *I can grow with you and know my own heart, mind, body, and soul. I can feel close to you and know yours.*

I wasn't reading any books on healing from abuse, but I don't think any of them would have recommended swiftly fall-ing in love and forging a lifelong union all within a year. Loving self first and taking the time to solidly know what you want before considering someone else's needs, especially a lover's, a new partner's—that's what I imagined the books would say. But my inner guidance didn't push these suggestions.

Maybe I did love myself already. Loving myself had given me the strength to leave. Loving myself was also a reason I stayed; I loved myself into staying alive in the relationship for as long as I could before I knew that leaving was the next best way to stay alive.

I knew how it felt to lose myself incrementally in smears and blurs, and now I knew how it felt to be moving closer to myself, every word, every choice. *No* felt like a heavy scuffle of hesitation, hiding, smallness, secrets, eyes cast down. And *yes* was becoming defined in opposition: soft center pulse of motion, dancing, expansive, truth spoken, eyes raised and ready.

I remembered who I was at fourteen years old when I refused to get confirmed in the Catholic Church because I had doubts and questions. *This will make Nana so sad,* my father said. But I wouldn't budge once I knew. *I can't confirm what I don't believe,* I declared. I loved myself in that moment too. It was with that same conviction that I knew that Lloyd and I could have a good life together. Deeply good. And that I wanted it. Believed in it. And believed in our courage to do the hard work of creating something new.

As snowflakes fall, different zones of temperature and slight changes of air moisture create layered patterns of water vapor as it freezes. Tossed by the wind, each snowflake experiences its own sequence, and its unique history imprints in its form. Moments it has passed through become crystallized and flash frozen. Unreturnable, singular instants. It's why no two snowflakes are identical.

We live like this. We heal like this too. On a different healing vector, I could have been led to a year abroad, teaching English in France and learning who I was abroad on my own. But I wasn't. That wasn't the life that animated me, even though I browsed those web pages. Healing was whatever felt right to return to life, to feel hope, to breathe in the cold morning air no matter what had been done to my body in nights before.

I was here in Jackson, hands making dragon body and dragon tail. Lloyd stacked and smoothed snow alongside me. We returned to the shoulders and added a thick neck that

rose a couple feet above our heads. We gathered sticks for
fangs and claws. We picked up fallen sweeps of pine brooms
to segment the tail. Here in Mississippi, my home, I held a
piece of ice against my lips and opened my mouth to taste.
The dragon mouth opened up to the white sky.

"I'm about to fuck up your gene pool," I joked, waving a
dragon claw at Lloyd. "Dominant traits incoming."

"Bring it on," he smiled, raising his hand for a snowy high
five. I'd been to his family reunion, where I stood in a buffet
line of blond heads and L. L. Bean vests. They even stood in
a circle facing each other in the sunshine and sang songs in
harmony like "I'll Fly Away." I didn't know families like this
actually existed outside of picture books.

In college I'd taken a Harlem Renaissance course and
was enthralled by Nella Larsen's novel *Passing*, in which a
biracial woman passes for white and marries a rich white
man. I'd never read about racial passing before, and though
I didn't vocalize its relevance to my own identity in class, I
began to develop a framework for myself. I could both be
fully accepted in white circles without question and yet when
I ordered a sandwich at Subway, the Black teenager behind
the counter asked me, *Tomato, lettuce, and onion?* in one
breath and *You mixed?* in the next. I'd also interviewed my
grandfather's brother, François, who told me that growing
up half-French in Cambodia, he never felt he belonged, but
then when he moved to Paris, he never fully belonged there
either and was treated as an outsider. Nana Jojo told me that
when her family evacuated to France after Algeria won its
independence, she was called *pied-noir*, or *black feet*, the
name given to those who were born and raised in Algeria

during colonial rule. She also grew up in a bilingual household, speaking French and Spanish since her mother was raised in Spain and her grandmother, who spoke only Spanish, lived with them. Even with these explorations, my racial reckoning still felt like my own private project.

I looked beyond the dragon toward the high fence on the west side of campus. In earlier decades the Midtown neighborhood near West Street had housed professors and students, but more recently, the community was made predominantly of people of color living at the poverty line. The institution did an about-face and shifted its entrance to the east side, the wealthier side, the whiter side. The college literally turned its back on the community.

This history was close to me as we constructed the dragon in view of Midtown because I was working with an initiative to build partnerships between the college and the Midtown community. I was learning from my mentor, the 1 Campus 1 Community director, Dr. Darby Ray, about what it meant to be in *partnership* as a community, rather than operating under the old community service model. Ideally, community partnerships are reciprocal and mutually transformative. About deep listening and collaboration, with a cultivation of relationships and distinctive strengths on each side.

Though I couldn't yet recognize it, my time with the program was rebuilding my perspective on my personal relationships, too, and who I was at my core. Not a broken girl in need of saving. Not a leech feeding on Lloyd's foundation of stability. Not an exotic outsider. Not a savior either. Lloyd brought one set of experiences, vulnerabilities, and possibilities, and I brought my own. I brought self-knowledge learned through mistakes, survival, listening, gold-fanged love, and the fire of an imagination determined to forge a new way. Just because my history held more recent generational trauma and the effects of an epidemic of violence against women didn't mean that I had less to offer. I'd lived in four regions of this country, and my family heritage spanned four continents in the last three generations. With a keen awareness of nuance and the ability to hold multiple complex truths of personal and social consciousness, I was just as much a culture shaper in our relationship as Lloyd. The defining factor wasn't only who J was versus who Lloyd was. It was about the effects we had on each other and who we became together. How we were inspired. What we co-created.

Still, I was actively resisting the idea that I was a messy girl full of baggage and drama. Because my history was living.

In early winter Dad had called me with some business about getting my tires rotated for free at Sam's Club and a receipt in the glove compartment. Then I heard a pause, a click of his mouth, the sound of the subject turning.

"Oh, and there was a letter in the mailbox for you. From J." I opened the envelope in the same way I felt the lump in my breast, needing to learn its size and its texture for my own health and safety. I held a single sheet of lined paper, folded in thirds to fit the envelope. J's handwriting marked the lines, measured and neat.

Dear Catherine, thank you. You have always been the catalyst for change I need in my life. I can now see that this situation is really no different. It didn't take me long to realize that your leaving was exactly what I needed. I needed a wake-up call. I know now what I must do to get my life back on track and to be the person you expect me to be. I won't bore you with empty promises of change, but I can promise that I am trying my hardest. A plan has already been set in motion to regain

control of my life. I'm seeing a counselor regularly, recon-
necting with old friends, and even starting the band again.
This has been a wonderful period of self-discovery for me.
It's going to take time, but I will show you that I am capable
of change. And just because you may not see or hear from
me doesn't mean that I've given up. I will be working hard
toward meeting my goals. I want to be the old me again. The
guy you fell in love with. I'm trying to not view this as a tragic
ending to our relationship but as a beautiful new beginning.
They say that some things in life are worth fighting for. You
are my first true love, Catherine. You are worth fighting for.
Until we meet again ... J

I hadn't heard his voice in writing or in person for almost
a year. It wasn't as sharp anymore, not a skewer. But it still
felt intimate, like my shirt taken off at the end of the day, still
warm from my body. I did not want this closeness.

I was glad to hear he was well. I still wanted a beautiful
new beginning for him. I did. Mostly I wanted whatever new
beginning would keep him from hurting another woman,
from hurting himself, from hurting me. I didn't want him to
rot in hell or live a lonely, miserable life. I didn't believe this
made me some highly evolved person or spiritually enlight-
ened; sometimes I thought I was a sucker for not being able
to call him a bad person. But I gulped a mixture of sadness,
anger, and fear to hear that he thought he was finding his way
back to me.

He thought we could have a future after what he did.

Worth fighting for. He had no awareness of my reality.
He had no idea that when I walked through a parking lot,
I felt safer seeing any random stranger than I would seeing
him. That every time I got in my car, I checked my back seat
to make sure he wasn't hiding there. That I still regularly

weighed whether I made the right decision in not filing charges, not for my own sense of justice but for preventing him from harming other women's bodies and futures. Maybe I'd made the wrong choice. He didn't realize the severity of what he'd committed. He could be in jail. He could be on the Sex Offender Registry. His crime could appear on background checks for employment. My jaw began to shake, and my lungs vibrated. I looked down and noticed my hands had lost their color, laced red with veins, my fingernail beds more purple than pink.

I slipped the letter back into the envelope and wondered if hearing from him meant I shouldn't go anywhere alone for a month. Could he work hard toward becoming the guy who left me alone? Could he work hard toward understanding why he chose to rape the woman he called his first true love? If I was worth fighting for, could he fight himself and his possessive instincts so that I could have my own beautiful new beginning, separate from him? Could he accept and believe that, above all, my own new beginning was what I deserved?

I want to be the old me again. The guy you fell in love with. He didn't realize that I wasn't the old *me* anymore. I wasn't the girl he fell in love with, and I never would be again. He may not even recognize the woman I've become.

Across days and into weeks the snow dragon stood. Long after the temperatures rose above freezing, after the ground snow melted, after the field sprang up green. The smallest mounds of tail melted first under the smile of the sun, while the largest pieces of the dragon's torso shrank day by day. Snow body small as a watermelon. *We created this.* Snow body small as an eggplant. *We created this.* Snow body small as a pomegranate. *We created this.* Snow body small as a fig. *We created this.* Eventually the grass drank the dragon fully. Even then I looked at the field and knew. *We're creating this.*

VAGINA ON FIRE

I text my midwife to see if we can meet for a pelvic exam. I say *hypergranulation*. I say *silver nitrate*. She says she'd be happy to see me. She gives me the address of a cottage she's renting to meet her pregnant clients in the Jackson area this weekend.

As I follow the map's route through the neighborhood by the airport, there is a pervasive Make America Great Again sign scowl furrowing the lawns. I try not to think about the headline I just read: *Trump administration "rolling back women's rights by 50 years" by changing definitions of domestic violence and sexual assault.* In their definition, domestic violence includes only physical harm, disregarding other forms of violence such as psychological harm, coercive control, and manipulation. This reduction rolls back years of research and awareness that abuse is more complex than a physical violence issue. It dismisses what I survived. The limited definition may also prevent victims from accessing essential support services.

I am a woman seeking respectful health care, I affirm as I drive. *I am a survivor tending to her body's wellness and making choices.* I haven't gone through everything in my past to suffer under the pressure of silence, to let doubts and questions fester. A person with a vulva and uterus should be able to tell the truth about their experiences and come out healthier, not sicker. That's what I drive toward.

Lydia opens the door for me with an apple-basket smile, and I step into a room that looks aggressively clean, recently flipped into butter-yellow gingham minimalist. More than I am nervous, I'm proud of myself for initiating this conversation. I have a list of talking points in a note on my phone, including *Is it possible I had a more severe tear?* and *Was there anything unusual about the repair?*

We chat, and I show her cute photos of the baby, and then I lie back on the queen bed. She shines a flashlight between my legs. She sees the scar tissue and uses the word *over-healing* just like my doctor did. Her voice has no alarm; she remembers nothing unusual about the repair. I was really swollen, she notes. Two layers tore, skin and muscle, and she sutured them both. Baby came out quickly once he crowned, while she applied a warm compress to my perineum to help prevent tearing.

All this makes sense. I don't know what I came to hear exactly; I wasn't looking for a loophole in her story that would unlock the mystery of my healing process. Maybe I needed to see what my body sensed in her presence, if I felt a red flag wave as we spoke. And I don't. She's the same person I trusted when I decided to birth with her.

I remember a moment in labor after I was fully dilated. *When do people usually take their underwear off? Is this a good time?* I called to her while I sat on the toilet and realized that maybe I didn't need to pull up my underwear because a baby would soon exit my vagina. *Well, what do you want to do?* she asked softly from the doorway. I tried to hand my power to her in that moment, and she handed it right back to me. I slipped my underwear off my ankles.

We say goodbye. Like a wind blowing in from another world, trust billows as I drive, and I want it. At my core, I have always wanted to trust. After J, that felt like naiveté. But I want to trust my intuition again. I don't need us to each play our part perfectly. I only need to know I can get in the mess with you and come out intact. The dead grass is blurring past me out the brown window, and I see a plane lifting to the sky. I think of my mother. How she was nineteen when she became a mother. How she spends her days entering the sky.

My parents met in South Florida in the reading room at the community college. Dad saw the tennis ball charm on my mom's keychain, which caught his attention since he was a competitive tennis player who trained with championship winners. He was wearing his classic '80s tennis shorts, side slit on his thick thighs, his brown hair flecked sun-gold blond. She'd just returned from a summer in Paris playing Elton John cassettes on her grandmother's balcony that bordered the Jardin du Luxembourg. He asked her if she wanted to get a coffee in the cafeteria, and she did.

Soon she met his family, and she fell in love with how quiet and peaceful his house felt, in contrast to the arguing and holdover-hippie parties at her own house. Before long they had matching disco outfits. She got pregnant, news that Nana recalls still with a keening of disbelief fresh in her voice—*No, Cathy, no.*

My parents swiftly married, and in 1982 my brother was born. Living with her in-laws, my mom cared for my brother full-time while my dad earned his bachelor's degree. He was in medical school by the time I was born in August 1987. I was a late baby, induced the week before my parents moved to Miami to be closer to the med school. Dad didn't want to know the sex of the baby, but when he stepped out of the room during the labor, my mom asked the nurse to tell her. *It's a girl*, the nurse whispered. *A girl*. Mom's eyes still get starry when she tells the story. The promise of a daughter carried her through the rest of the twenty-four-hour birth.

Shortly after our family moved to Mississippi, right before my first period, my mother went away for six weeks to train to be a flight attendant. *I've given everything to you kids for over fifteen years. I need to do something for myself*, she said. I knew it was true; I could feel my mother's longing to fly. I wanted her to have it. I helped her study her training manuals, memorizing scripts for emergency evacuations and water landings. We laughed as I signaled the exits with my forefingers waving to the front, back, and sides of our invisible aircrafts. I remember believing that I was a good child because I was supportive and I understood her needs. If I gave her my blessing to go, it would honor all that she had given to us, to me.

The azaleas have flamed. At our house and all across the city, spring is a torch. I drive the kids to our old college campus, where at the center, a garden burns red and pink. Guider picks off a pink blaze and grinds the petals into the sidewalk with his fingertip. He reaches for another flower and a stick. He pulls the petals apart, rolls them between his fingers, and tosses them to the concrete, scratching the fibers to smithereens with the stick.

"I'm drilling flowers!" he announces, stomping back to the bush. If ever there were a time for me to think, *all boy!* this would be it. *All boy* means playing in the dirt, making weapons out of sticks, and being wild in a distinctly masculine way that looks for a fight and a challenge. *All boy* means being drawn to action rather than feelings, with the will to conquer. It means moving through the world like a little tornado that makes messes and laughs in its wake. This phrase, said as a warning with an affectionate smile by mothers, church aunties, and proud fathers—*He's all boy!*—has been known to burn right through me like a sentencing.

I remember a moment earlier this week: I am trying to cushion Guider's head in my hands while he broncos against the tile. I gap my belly out of the target line of his kicking feet and say to myself, *Big feelings, I can hold space for his big feelings.* Inside my cells spin chaotically with the past, memories of holding J when he spiraled, hurting me and seeking my comfort like two wings of the same dying butterfly.

A scream wedges under my clavicle, and I'm trapped here at the bony joints. Part of me wants to squeeze my fingers as tight as I can around my son's arms and shout at him to snap out of it. Heat pools in my mouth, daring me to unleash a power I could never use before. There she is, Hungry Wraith Girl, who buried her rage and her fight so she could survive. As my son grows more willful, less baby, this wraith girl gets hungrier in her graveyard, as if she wants something between justice and revenge. It's her world now, not the boys'.

This is your two-year-old, I remind myself. *Not a grown man.* He needs space to release his anger so it doesn't get alloyed into weapons used against himself and others. My hands cup his banging head; my knuckles knock against the floor. On my knees I wait it out as my spit warms in my mouth. I remember to breathe, but even my breath remembers the dead.

Eventually it ends.

When I tell Kristen about the way this moment pinned me, she says, "Wow, J really acted like a toddler, didn't he?" Her voice is so casual that it thins the weight of the air. A sound deep in my throat, not quite laughter.

I had a boyfriend who acted like a child. Now when my toddler acts like a toddler, I see a boyfriend.

A flash of sheen from the azaleas catches the sun and brings me back to this garden. I take a closer look at a pink blossom still on the stem. I turn the flower, and milky stripes glisten in the light. The flecks, almost opalescent, look like my stretch marks, more visible after this second baby. I see us everywhere now: signs of the mother. The strength of women shimmers down my spine like a snake tail. How many of us were asked to exert our caregiving energy before we were even grown? Raising ourselves, raising our siblings, parenting our parents, mothering our boyfriends. By the time we become mothers, we're already exhausted. Care work is a sinister swarm.

Compared with my mom, I'd had almost ten more years of life before I became a mother, twenty-eight to her nineteen. I pursued an advanced degree and earning power, found more confidence in my voice and my relationships, learned about what I wanted, and advocated for my needs. I thought that extra decade would mean that I wouldn't arrive at motherhood grieving the lost opportunity to develop myself first, how my mother felt. But in motherhood I have still felt *an aching feeling that I am losing myself.* The same words I wrote as a seventeen-year-old when I dated J. I couldn't protect myself from that aching loss, and it reminds me of how I couldn't protect myself from a toxic, abusive relationship even after studying my mom's and nana's turbulent marriages. They struggled financially and emotionally after their divorces, after they'd given so much of themselves to their families. In the end, they were treated as if their care was a basic, expected part of the marriage bargain, not highly skilled and valuable free labor, not their very brilliance. I'm angry for them. And I'm bursting with new appreciation for what they gave us.

I want to hug every mother on the planet.

Guider spins the stick atop the flower mound on the pavement. Then he stands, and his fingers fly through the air slowly. I see that nestled between his fingers is a pink blossom, still intact.

"They're trying to become butterflies," he whirrs.

Under dropped ceiling fluorescence, Veronica and I sit down by the computer, where she asks me pages of questions she calls The Sexual Function Index.

How often do you have an orgasm? How strong would you rate your orgasm?

How difficult is it for wetness to occur? And does it last for the entire sexual activity?

What kind of masturbation do you do?

How do you feel about the emotional connection with your partner during sex?

Do you guide your partner's penis in for entry?

How often do you feel aroused?

I tell her things I've never told my friends. I tell her things I've never told my doctor. I tell her things I've never told Lloyd. Nor myself. It's a soft landing; we're sitting on the moss couch. We talk for more than an hour, until my breasts swell with my baby's next meal. We talk until I feel my nipples tingle and my bra dampen.

Veronica encourages me to set the intention for intimacy whenever I'm ready, in order to help prepare emotionally and physically. "For example, you might send him a text that says, 'Hey, I want to see you in the bedroom tonight [wink].'"

I leave before my milk spills through my shirt.

I don't really want to see him in the bedroom tonight, not in the cute winking way, but I want something new, something different, a new story for us.

"I am ever so respectfully lusting after you," Lloyd whispers to me when he passes me in the hallway before bed. I flash my Lady Gray eyes at him. I have been feeling surges of desire on my own. More than I've felt in years. On a couple nights we've made out like teenagers with our underwear on, rubbing and gripping and releasing. When my orgasm hits the crest of the wave, milk spills from me and becomes a slick warmth between our chests. My milk feels kinky in a way I didn't choose. But here it is, bard of an ancient tale of oxytocin, the bonding hormone that connects sex, birth, and breastfeeding. *No part of you is separate*, the milk seems to wink at me, a bawdy trickster.

We lie next to each other in bed. Lloyd strokes my hair, and I study his face, trying to really see him. My eyes travel up to that one swooping eyebrow hair and then down to the blond fringe peeking out of his nostrils. Here is my love, my partner. Yesterday I sent him a picture of our first child's poop in the lime-green bowl of the toddler potty. He called us from work to celebrate, a swan song to diapers. The last text from him contained five words: *Out running. Back by 8:30.* Now we emerge from this density of parenthood, as if searching for two stars in a heavily clouded sky, trusting that they still burn. It feels radical that we're choosing something other than sleep. *Love, come find me.*

His lips brush my areolas, and I invite him on top of me naked, with the qualification that this won't be sex as we know it, no artistic liberties please. This will be a study of new body mechanics: just follow my directions and move slower than slow. He sits at my entrance, dutiful, and I feel the pressure of his hardness, warm on the flaming pearl and silken with coconut oil. Rather than trying to probe past pain with the wedge of my hands, I take my hands away and tell him to stay totally still. I breathe around him, each inhale naturally pulling him a little closer and each exhale slowly releasing the pressure. We don't talk. We are silent like meditation. My vagina guides him, guides me. When I exhale, I relax my pelvic floor muscles and the space between us becomes shorter. It's the same way that I breathed my baby down and out.

Once he's more inside than out, I feel each of his breaths like a twinge of pulpy sharpness. I caution a shallow squeeze with my pelvic muscles. He gently taps back. I ask him to rest there for a minute with nothing moving but our breath. My body does not sing with sensations of pleasure. But even singers honor measures of rest, counting the beats until their next note vibrates from them, strong and true.

April begins. I return to the gynecologist. We've waited six weeks between the silver nitrate treatments to see how the tissue would respond to more spacing. Our answer: not well. Not only has the scar tissue not retreated but it has regrown, even larger. Long, pink flesh petals fall in my valley.

Even though the news is not good, I can't help but respect my body's dogged healing. It may not be healing in the direction we wanted, but its effort makes me want to wrap my arms around the wound, cradle it, and say, *Hey, I see you trying.*

When my doctor applies the silver nitrate, the burning smolders down to the roots. The scars feel more alive, like the first time. *Coat the healthy tissue with Vaseline; keep the flesh around it safe.* After, I open the drawer for a panty liner and squeeze my thighs together so the liquid wax won't drip down my leg.

Once I'm dressed, she comes back in to talk. We thought we'd be finished with the treatments by now. Three or four she had originally expected. This was number five. I'll need at least two more, she's telling me. Her words come down like a hatchet. I nod, swallowing a lump. Tears remain moist clouds in my ducts. I want this to end. I want to know that healing ends.

"This is not a significant issue in the medical world," she assures me, as in, *We are handling this. We can fix this.* But she quickly reaches for a handout and clarifies, "It's not significant in severity. But that doesn't mean it's insignificant to you."

When I leave, I drive to a conference room where Lloyd and I are meeting our financial advisor. As soon as I sit in the conference chair, my pelvis feels incendiary. I get shifty in my seat, trying to balance the pressure. I find that it's most comfortable to lean back in a *man spread*, in which I coax a pocket of air between my labia so the burning doesn't kiss at the center. This puts me in a lazy listener posture, but if I lean forward, I feed the fire. I try to train my eyes on the wall monitor with the calculations, but my vagina feels like a mile-long driveway of fresh hot tar in front of me. I muster friendliness and coherence while my voice pinches into a flighty tenor. I wonder how many women are muscling through boardrooms at this very moment with ferocious postpartum flesh texturing their words. What would we give if we really understood what a mother's body has given? A voice makes strips of my tongue and seethes, *We would give her everything*.

Once home, I open the door with a smile and overenthusiastic hellos. The sight of me makes Rowan vocalize and begin grunting for milk. He wants The Mama. I wave *I'll be right back* and tousle Guider's hair as I rush to the bathroom. I already know I will be relying heavily on *CoComelon* the rest of the day.

By now, my whole vulva is a pouch of lava. I close the window shutters, pull down my leggings, and grab the hand mirror. I bend my knees and look.

My inner labia flame raw, as if peeled down to a layer closer to my blood. Something has gone wrong. The burning spread from my insides to the outside. Did the silver nitrate melt into the Vaseline, seeping out? I go dizzy at the sight as I bend over. I reach out my hands to steady myself against the counter. My fingers tremble, and my stomach flicks like a fish tail.

Something raw and ancient reawakens with this flesh burn. The bones of old stories want me to scavenge them again, to slide my teeth against their dry shards and gnaw off any edible shreds. On the worst days, like today, my vagina tells me that suffering will always be my work, my feminine inheritance. My whole self feels *made to withstand trauma.*

I hear Rowan beginning to cry from the other side of the house. I'm full of milk, but already I feel sucked dry.

I feel it happening again. The Martyr Mother wants me to follow her to a bitter place, to sacrifice her own needs for everyone else's. Inside her lives the Hungry Wraith Girl too. They say, *This pain is your place in the world. You thought you would be the first generation to break away and be free, but you won't. This is just how it is to be a woman, to be a mother.*

If I stay with the Martyr Mother, I get to stay with my own mother and my grandmother, and we can stew together in all our sacrifices. We'll speak a common language of missed opportunities, overworked wounds, and feeding everyone else while we forget we're hungry.

If I leave the Martyr Mother behind, I feel as if I'm abandoning the women I love who came before me, as if I'm leaving home for good and moving to a new land with a new language from the mother tongue, where our common words and feelings will become smaller and smaller.

Who do you think you are that you get to want more? the Martyr Mother asks. But whose voice is it anyway?

It's not my nana's voice that I heard when she showed up in my doorway at midnight while I studied to say, "Catherine, go to bed. You need your rest." It's not my mother's voice, the one that says, "Sweetie, you're brilliant. You can do anything."

It's time to leave the bathroom.

Designed to stretch and tear and return to a healthy state. That's the other part of what Dr. S told me. I've stretched,

I've torn, I've burned. When I stand, I want to know that I'll do whatever it takes to walk toward the healthy state. And that in cultivating health, caring for myself, I'm not abandoning my foremothers in their pain but honoring them. I want to walk toward what's next for us, for all of us.

PART THREE

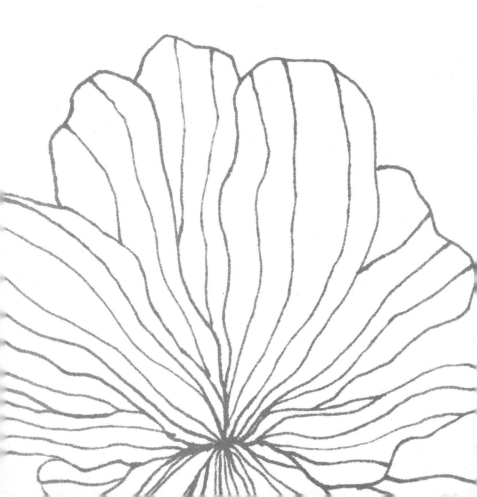

SPEAK, THOU
CLITORIS

When my milk arrived months earlier, it spilled from me. Every time I stepped out of the shower, my breasts, having been pelted by the water's heat, dripped a steady tap of white beads. They fell like blood. An army of sugar ants arrived for the food that poured from me and dried into flakes of creamy milk crystals on the floor. Suddenly my body's compulsion was creation, regeneration, fuel. The creative force pressed into me even more urgently than in pregnancy. The word *milkshed* began cycling in my mind, like a sister to *bloodshed*.

Pleasure arrived in the same way, a loud sister to the pain of my scars.

I wake up one morning with a strong directive of desire from my body. Not for sex, but for something new. My skin feels loose and oversized, leaky and formless, spilling over. I want to be pressed, squeezed, with my flesh pushing against seams. A craving for tight resistance. The story I've told myself for a long time is that I prioritize comfort over appearances, which has meant stretchy leggings and flowy tunics. But today the spaciousness isn't comfortable; it's unsettling. I went hard and taut in my skin in gestation. But when my baby left my belly, I became slack, like a rope between two hands that droops onto the floor. *Where does my body end?* So much energy flows out through my milk; my breasts seem to end in my baby's mouth, even when he's across the house. I tingle at the sound of his cry and then Guider hangs on my leg, tugging at my skirt, and I feel endless.

Before I got pregnant with Rowan, Kristen had given me the assignment to notice moments of desire in my day. To simply notice if I felt turned on. To do something that felt sexy just for myself, like wearing lingerie under my clothes.

"Have you ever just worn a thong because you liked the way it felt?" Kristen offered as an example. My mom's laundry basket was always decorated with thongs that twisted like curled, dried bamboo leaves. I thought women wore thongs for sex appeal and to hide their panty line; and after my teens, I wasn't invested in either one, so I decided it wasn't for me. "Well, it doesn't have to be a thong. It can be anything that feels good against your skin and that makes you walk around feeling confident or that makes you notice your libido," Kristen said. I sat there knowing that under my clothing was my nursing bra with circles of milk stained like tree rings and cheap cotton underwear sold in packs of six.

But today I have a desire, just for myself. I follow it to my closet, where my hands find a woven basket and a thong I wasn't sure was still there. My fingers trace black lace. I hike the thong up my thighs, and the strappy sides make divots in my hips. Yes. Relief. I dig deeper into the basket and there's a push-up bra, burlesque red with a wing of black lace. I loop my arms through and fasten the clasp. The bra holds me, and the thong hugs. Yes. I am close to satisfying my body's urges. But I crave even more structure.

In the same corner of the closet, I find the striped, woven rebozo that I used in birth. Cassandra, my childbirth teacher, had taught me how to wrap the scarf snugly around my belly, cross it behind my back, and grasp the ends over my shoulders. The rebozo could make a container for the contractions, showing me where the strong sensations ended and reminding me that my body held the force of it all. *You are bigger than the sensations.* The pain didn't come from *outside* of me but from deep within me. During contractions, I'd leaned forward on the toilet while gripping the tasseled ends of the rebozo. I could cup the pain, squeeze it, and contain it until the contraction warmed like clay in my hands.

Over the thong and the underwire bra, I wrap the rebozo around my middle and I tie myself in. Just as in birth, the counterpressure feels good. I know where my skin ends and everything else begins.

When a cicada emerges from the ground as a nymph, it climbs the first surface it finds and sloughs off its exoskeleton to begin its final transformation into adulthood. An exoskeleton cannot stretch; it must be discarded in order for the animal to grow. Filling itself with water or air to crack the too-small outer shell along weak points, the animal struggles to free itself from the old encasement. Once free, the cicada, soft and vulnerable inside its new, unhardened skeleton, unfolds its crumpled wings.

I gaze out the window past the forest-green walls into a landscape of herons, possums, and beavers. The Pearl River and bald cypress swamps are just out of sight. I've dropped the kids off at Lloyd's work during his lunch break so I can attend my weekly therapy session. Most of my hours away from my children are earmarked for physical or emotional healing these days. PT, silver nitrate, therapy, repeat. Kristen sits across from me in an armchair.

"I want to know that healing ends. I want healing to be a story with a beginning, a middle, and an end," I tell her, exhausted.

"What would it feel like to be healed?" she asks, curiosity rising.

I've never considered this before. Healing has been a vanishing horizon line. How would I even know if I've arrived there? Even if it's a lifelong process, surely there are different milestones along the way.

"I guess to feel that I'm aware of the past wound—I don't pretend it's not there—but it doesn't hurt so much that it prevents me from doing what's important to me. I'm no longer making decisions from a wounded place."

"What would it *look* like to be healed?" she asks. Her eyes are bright, glint of the wild woman.

In the car, hanging onto the moments of quiet before I drive back to my kids, I scribble the first words that come to me: *I could confidently request how I want to be touched. I would feel adventurous, bold, and playful in my body. I wouldn't find it too intense to look in my partner's eyes when making love. I wouldn't fear losing control. I wouldn't feel ashamed to vocalize when I experience pleasure. I can see her: free, expressive, assertive, passionate.*

Spring begins flirting with Mississippi, pollen coating our cars in thick layers. Morgan suggests I listen to a podcast called *Thirst Aid Kit*. I turn it on while I'm in the bathtub, and I immediately warm to the voices of Nichole Perkins and Bim Adewunmi, two women who are unapologetic and confident in their sexual thirst. They say things like, *I bet he mashes his cornbread in his greens, eats it with his fingers, then looks at you like "You next."* I smile. It's not the usual fare of sexy bodies I've known, all muscle and grind. They notice how a man's voice—*a pressure in the back of his throat, how he grits his teeth*—sparks their attraction. I haven't realized just how parched my erotic imagination has been until I hear their vivid imaginings about bodies.

Soon after, while driving home from yoga, I hear a woman on public radio describing the kinds of biscuits she likes to eat. *I want a sturdy biscuit. Flaky with a durable bottom. I want my teeth to leave marks in it. I want it to be able to withstand gravy and keep its form.*

It's a cooking show, but after listening to Nichole and Bim and now this biscuit lover, I find myself thinking, *Damn, I want to be able to describe the way I like being touched that way.* Before long, I'm typing comments about Lloyd in my phone notes that make me smile. *His butt is understated, firm as two frozen biscuits. He rises, he rises, he rises with heat.* Even though Lloyd and I have both memorized the first lines of the prologue of *The Canterbury Tales* in Middle English and are constant communicators, I still feel shy and guarded when talking about sex.

The truth is that the vibration of sex in my throat and mouth has felt too vulnerable for years. Early on, I used moaning as a way to hasten unwanted sex, and ever since, the sounds have felt like performance. And communication about sex felt dangerous. My mouth once filled with *no* and *stop* before it was filled with an organ I didn't want there. I have a hunch that for a long time, maybe the rest of my life, the answer to *What's the worst thing that's ever happened to you?* will be this violence that happened in my mouth.

Ever since, sex has felt truer in my silence, and pleasure is a hard candy savored in my cheek pocket. I flick it across my tongue and it melts, my own.

But my mind keeps returning to birth, when I moaned wildly and freely. Bass tones, gravity sounds, down down down. Moaning was a cave I let the pain vibrate through, a place to cup the intensity when I couldn't run from it. And just the other day when I lowered myself into the hot bath, an *ahhh* steamed from me. I want sex to feel how music feels in my body.

Vibrations in my throat, vibrations across the skin bridge. When a relationship has operated within unnamed rules for years, those laws of motion live inside you. Objects in motion stay in motion. Objects at rest stay at rest. But my body will not stay at rest.

The baby monitor is silent, and I'm ready to ask Lloyd to join me in my explorations.

"I've been noticing that my body responds differently to touch since birth," I tell him, cheek on my pillow. "Will you try something new with me?" He's curious and ready.

I ask him to firmly press and tap my butt with a flat palm. Flex handed, he starts slapping lightly.

"Over here," I demonstrate. "I'm trying to figure out where it feels best and what level of pressure." He tries tapping over the crevice of my butt cheeks, then lower toward my labia, to the right and then to the left. Sometimes more staccato and other times a lingering pressure. "Yeah, that's a good spot. A little firmer there. Try that faster," I say neutrally, as if guiding him to position a painting on the wall.

I never thought this would be something I would ask for. At first I'm a little uneasy. *Am I the kind of person who likes to be spanked now?* When I'd seen this in movies before, it had been accompanied with leather straps and bondage, and I thought the point was pleasure in pain. But that doesn't match what I am experiencing. This feels gentle, wind chimes singing between my legs. I suspend the story and track what my body tells me.

His hands move up my back, where I feel a knot I want released.

"Run your fingers along my shoulder blade. Yeah, now press there." The natural impulse to make a sound of relief pushes up my throat. A quiet moan buzzes in my closed mouth. I let it out.

"Would you practice something with me? I'm going to play with some sounds here. Would you make some pleasure sounds, too?"

I release my jaw and clip a low moan from my throat, let it fall out, let its petals scatter around me. Hum, grunt, low growl, air dreaming of air. Something happens. Rather than the memory of using moans to speed up sex in J's room with screensaver tessellations, I see myself in this bedroom six months prior, laboring with these sounds. *Good, that's so good,* I hear my midwife say.

"Would you make some of those low, rumbling growl sounds that you make when things get intense for you?" Sometimes his sex sounds make my chest tighten with panic that his pleasure might spiral out of control. But right now I know who we are, and I'm not afraid. I want to approach the edges of my discomfort to make new associations. Triggers, like scars, can be lovingly touched.

His voice ripples down to his lower scales, into primal resonance.

I am safe. I choose this. I am safe. I breathe space around the urge to tighten, recoil, or float away. I stay with his fingers brushing my ribcage, tracing the wings of my bird. I stay with each moan. As his hands start to travel back down to my rear, I hear a *no* from my body, throat tightening in alert, too much too soon.

"Not there. Touch my back. I want to normalize your sounds while you're touching somewhere that doesn't feel so emotionally charged for me."

His fingers shine my shoulder blades again, so tight they feel rusted shut. For hours each day I hunch over our nursing baby and keep my watch downward at our toddler, eyes always accounting *what's in his hands, what's in his mouth, where is he going next?*

I know what it is to be *touched out*, swarming with fingers pinching my neck mole and hands swerving toward my breasts as handlebars. But tonight I am touched in. I don't want to crawl out of my skin; I want to crawl in deeper.

hummingbird migration

Three hours north of Jackson, almost all the way to Memphis, sits the small town of Holly Springs. Lloyd and I began our marriage in a small brick house on Cedar Drive.

"This is more Mississippi than I've ever known," I declared. This meant the town was a food desert. This meant that its tiny population had produced thirteen Confederate generals. This meant that one day I had an impulse to search the local Sex Offender Registry, and only a few last names were unfamiliar from the rosters where I taught sixth-grade English.

In the Mississippi Teacher Corps, I was placed in a critical needs school in the even more rural town of Byhalia, where 98 percent of the kids were enrolled in free and reduced-price lunch. When the new corps of teachers arrived, the director of the program made me straighten in my seat with this greeting: "You shouldn't be here. The most experienced teachers in the country should be in the most challenging schools. But they won't come here. So here we are."

I still needed to prove to myself that I was not too sensitive and yielding for this world. I wanted the muscle of a teacher voice, a voice of confidence and leadership. I wanted to become that voice. In training, we were taught not to smile in the first month of the school year. We were taught to practice looking in the mirror while asserting, *no, warning, copy assignment, detention.*

My classroom was between the old football locker room and the parking lot dumpster, where kids flung each other's backpacks; they hid behind the parked cars if I didn't usher them into the classroom quickly enough. From the moment my students arrived in the morning, I began de-escalating arguments with catapulting insults like *You a big pinto bean head* and *Don't make me go ham* (hard as a motherfucker).

Lloyd packed my lunches in the morning, crafting peanut butter sandwiches with surprises in the middle like coconut shavings, a cluster of chocolate chips, or a single dried apricot. While I had appreciated his whimsy in the fro-yo cones he crafted for me in college, now I had an onslaught of stimuli, too many layers of sight and sound to process.

"I love that you make my lunch. But please just make me something boring," I told him. "No surprises. The last thing I need is a sandwich that confronts my senses."

In the evening he tried to make me laugh with comedic bebop rhymes and the Billy Bob Thornton *Sling Blade* voice, but I'd been churning in the loud antics of middle school hallways since daybreak, always a preteen cackling or rubbing a burn by saying, *Ooooo, she feeeeelin' it.*

My skin vibrated with the day long after I swept the last empty hot sauce packet off my classroom tiles. As I drove home, the next day's sound already queued up in my body, like a subcutaneous playlist on repeat. Pencils falling, pencils cracking, pencils electrically sharpened to the point of split lead. A boy bragging about the dogfights he had watched over the weekend. A crumpled note on my floor that said: *Mrs. Gray is a bitch and she can suck my dick.* By evening, I only wanted to sink into the dull reverie of *Law and Order: SVU*, with episodic pain of a more heinous nature than I'd witnessed that day.

"I thought I would be good at supporting kids in tough situations because I've always been a good listener and able to build trust with people," I told Lloyd while we sat in the kitchen eating the spaghetti he had made. "But I feel like I've been at an emotional rock concert all day, like the speakers have been right next to my ears for hours. It's deafening. I feel like I'm failing them, like I want to be able to give my full attention to the kid standing in front of me, but my attention is always being pulled to the next thing. I don't even feel like a good listener anymore."

"I know you're trying so hard," Lloyd said. "I can see how much it matters to you to do a good job. I bet you're making more of an impact than you think you are."

He saw me as stronger than I knew I was. *Steel wrapped in cotton,* he called me. Upright and tall in my demeanor despite all I had been through. Persistent in my soft welcome.

I turned off the light in bed, and Lloyd's palm made circles on my shoulder blades.

"I miss you," he said. I blinked in darkness. I understood it was my body he was missing, our bodies together. I calculated seven hours of sleep available before my alarm went off at 5 a.m. Those were hours of unconsciousness that I wanted. Desire? It felt as if my body had been emptied of that furniture, yearning instead for silence and space. No one needing me. No one asking for me. No one edging so close that

I could smell their sweat glands. I didn't want to be a cliché of sex dying after marriage, but I also had a more intimate physical relationship with my saline sinus rinse.

I could feel the vulnerability in his voice, reaching for me. I didn't want him to feel rejected or undesirable. Not my new husband who moved to this brain-drain town, three hours from our friends and the field where we built the snow dragon, all so I could teach and earn a free master's degree while he took slurred orders for honey-gold hot wings at Michael's Country and Creole. Sometimes there's nothing scarier than a person missing you when you're right beside them.

So I tried.

After our bodies met, after our bodies parted and he rolled out of bed to the bathroom, I inhaled deeply. An empty square dropped in my chest, something like sadness bordered with loneliness. A feeling that had no color, like an empty cellophane bag. As if sex was something done to me. *Never again*, I promised myself.

"I'm trying to protect us," I told him on another night in bed. "I know what it feels like to say *yes* when I don't really want sex. I felt it the other night—I don't know, I guess, empty. But I didn't know how I was feeling until after. I don't want that to become normal."

He didn't want that for me or for us either. But I also saw confusion in his eyes about how far away my body had suddenly become. I got undressed in the bathroom with the door closed. *My stomach hurts*, I mentioned as we brushed our teeth, a preemptive decline of a bid. When I got into bed, I turned my back to him.

He still thought he could help me want our naked bodies breathing into each other, as a comfort, as a relief, as a sparkler of fun available to us even here in this spoiled-milk town. A squeeze of my hips, and fingertips circling down my vertebrae. Lips on the side of my neck. I wanted to want it. Or I wanted to *want* to want it. Sex had been surprisingly easy and wildflower-lush for awhile, as if I'd never been hurt.

He stroked my hair, but his fingers got tangled in my curls, and I flinched.

Since childhood, my body had been a holding place for my pain so that when someone said, *Where does it hurt?* I could say, *Here.* And if I kept noticing pain, I could keep pointing to places.

It began in fourth grade with the migraines. Throbbing in my head, pulsing behind my eyes. My white-haired teacher Mrs. Gommels handed us a stack of worksheets in the morning, and she scowled at me from her desk when I worked too slowly. At the same time, home became shaky. I started to sense shifts in my family. Mom was changing. Her shirts got tighter and stretchier, and she began spending hours in the basement on our computer, dialing up to chat rooms and smiling at something outside of our life. Dad drove me around Iowa City while jazz radio trilled in his jerky, stick-shift Corolla. For years I would think that jazz made me sick, an imprecise nausea linked to saxophones, exhaust fumes, and summer humidity.

That year insomnia hit. A deep dread weighed in my gut when bedtime came, and when I did fall asleep, the pulsing in my head woke me. In the middle of the night, I sat on my shag carpet and drank mugs of Sleepytime tea while the imagist

French film *Le ballon rouge* flashed in the dark. Laughter, carousel wheels turning, faint voices of French schoolchildren. One red balloon floated across the misty City of Lights, always just out of the schoolboy's friendly reach.

My body could say things that my voice couldn't, truths I wasn't ready to understand.

Bedtime was becoming a dreaded event again, attached to feeling like a bad wife for lacking interest in sex during what was supposed to be *our honeymoon phase*. A reminder that falling asleep meant waking up to go back to school. Sometimes I fantasized about getting pregnant so I would have a good reason to quit the teaching program, although I knew that was no reason to have a baby.

Lloyd sat on the floor next to me while I lay on the couch. He rested two fingers on my neck to track my pulse while he looked down at his watch. "135," he said, after a thirty-second sample. His heart hit that rate only when he was running. He counted again, waiting thirty more seconds. Again, 135. Almost twice as fast as the average resting heart rate. I could hear my heart in my ears, and each beat felt heavy, like a ruby-throated hummingbird inside a wire cage.

In Holly Springs, we lived in the corridor of the hummingbird migration. In September, hundreds of hummingbirds thickened the sky, darting and diving for the nectar that would sustain them. We'd watched tiny bands get attached to their legs, to track their physical condition and the impact of habitat loss.

After rest on the couch and no improvement in my heart rate, we called my dad, who told us to drive to a hospital. Soon I would be admitted, where an EKG would show a condition I'd never had before: a right bundle branch block in my heart. An electrical issue. My right ventricle was not perfectly in sync with the left. This matched what I sensed, the sensation that my heart limped with one foot dragging behind it.

I took a week off school to rest, maxing out my sick days. I was grateful I had an urgent reason to take a break, although I never said this aloud. My body set limits that I wasn't willing to voice.

My cardiologist never found any more answers to what caused the condition. "Stress?" and a shoulder shrug seemed to be the best answer we had. "You have a very robust sympathetic nervous system," he added. A robust fight-or-flight response. He made it sound like a compliment, but it reminded me of something my ophthalmologist had recently said: "You have very active eyes." Eyes that move quickly and often. Eyes that scan for threat. Nerves that send impulses to the brain that say: *You are not safe.*

Still, I didn't connect these issues to anything beyond the stress of teaching.

It was January, a Monday. I was sitting under my down comforter with my laptop leaking my *dark and cerebral* recommendations curated by Netflix. In between episodes, I opened Facebook and saw I had a DM from a woman whose name I already knew, though I'd never met her. Holding my breath, I opened her message.

You probably don't know who I am. And this is kind of weird that I know who you are . . . I'm writing you about J. The truth is that I've wanted to talk to you for a while now, but the past few months have been the most worrisome, dramatic, and scary. I want to know what kind of things J did after you two broke up. If you don't want to read any further or answer me, just ignore this message and I will understand.

The suspicious part of me fueled by true crime and my dad's school of self-defensive daughters kicked in first. *Was it possible that J was putting her up to this? Would she show my words to him?* It was years before the *Believe women* slogan, but once those initial questions flared, I knew how to believe Meredith better than I knew how not to. I didn't want to live in a world where I wouldn't believe a woman, a fellow girlfriend of J, reaching out to me for help. If I was wrong to trust her, well, call me that fool.

When I'd first found out they were dating, I'd wondered if I should warn her. But I hoped that J could change; mutual friends said he was doing well. Maybe we just had a particularly toxic effect on each other. My stomach twisted now. He was still hurting women.

My heart raced as I typed my story in response. His jealousy, possessiveness, and his controlling grasp. His suicide threats if I left him. My isolation from my friends and family. The rape. My escape. His stalking. As I typed, it occurred to me that I'd never written the story of what happened over those four years. I shared my feelings, too: *I didn't want to abandon someone I loved while he was suffering, but I couldn't quite see how bad it was while I was in it.*

At the end I said: *I still have nightmares about J. I worry that one day he will try to find me. I don't know when and if I'll ever stop being afraid. It's always in the back of my mind.*

Meredith wrote back an hour later. Immediately we recognized patterns. One night when she was visiting friends out of town, he called her at 3 a.m. a total of fifty times with voicemails to match, each one becoming more insulting and hurtful. He told both of us we should be thankful he wasn't worse. We both feared for our loved ones and felt we needed to move out of the city, the state, or even the region to be safe. She had moved to New York City.

Over the next week we wrote more than six thousand words to each other. I had told friends about J's concerning behavior, the insults, and my fear, but it felt different when I wrote to Meredith. We were surviving the same person, and she wasn't free of him yet. He was still making new email addresses every time she blocked him. We both knew the exact crazy way that J's eyes looked when he cornered us in public. We both knew this war of self-conservation that she described:

> *i think i would feel a lot better about life, oddly enough, if*
> *i just wanted him to suffer. isn't that backwards? because*
> *whenever i want him to be ok, i want to help him. and that's*
> *just the start of another bad cycle.*

I gave her my phone number, but she never called. We only messaged through our fingers, reading the words in our own voices. Maybe she jumped every time the phone rang like I did, beating wings so fast they were almost invisible. Maybe she learned to keep her phone on silent. Maybe we each needed to witness the words on our screens, artifacts of abuse that stayed invisible.

We didn't call it *abuse*. I called it *this mess*. She called it *this situation*.

Wish you the best! she wrote before we each flew away.

THE VULVA
PORTRAITS

I step out of the shower, towel myself, and recline on the bed. I open my legs and rest the jar next to me, spooning a small pat of coconut oil that melts into slick-shine on my fingers. Then I greet the familiar spots: the bead of scar tissue at the lip, the firm ribbon that unspools inside, the skin bridge on my perineum.

I see Lloyd's form in the doorway in his pj pants and T-shirt. I'm not wearing my glasses, so his expression blurs.

"I'm massaging scar tissue," I explain.

"As a young man I was taught that if a lady was naked on the bed looking in my direction with her hands on her genitals, that this portended well for sex for that night. I have to amend my associations," he smirks.

On the spot I decide that there *is* something I want from him.

"You said awhile back that you didn't like to look at my vulva very much. I think that part of what's happening is that you haven't gotten to know it." I realized my responsibility in this too. I didn't like him to look or touch over the years because the vulnerability seared me; I'd pushed him away so many times that he had stopped asking.

"A vulva is not like a penis," I continue. "It's not just hanging around on the outside. You won't know it unless we make intentional time for you to do that." I swallow to summon my courage, my directness. "I'd like you to draw my vulva."

His mouth tugs to the side like it does when he's nervous, bracing against the pull to shut down. I see him working to stay soft, *to love* as a verb. Determining if he can say *yes* as a choice rather than an assignment. I feel my own fear that I'm controlling and have all the power, having defined so many terms of our intimacy that he's respected; and now I'm asking him to do a vulnerable new thing after years of operating within the narrow lines of my comfort.

"I'm not asking for a masterpiece," I qualify, knowing his painting classes and his perfectionism. "I'm not worried about the product or how you'll interpret my vulva on the page. It can be very impressionistic. It can be four lines. I think this may be a good way for you to get to know my genitals."

"Okay," he surrenders, even though exhaustion flumes his voice. I sense his fear of sleep scarcity; his eyelids usually get heavy around 10 p.m. while my irises are just starting to glisten.

He finds the pen and notebook and moves to my feet.

"Should I—"

"This will be easier if you don't talk," he interjects. I hear a boundary; he'll draw my vulva like I asked, but that's his max capacity right now. No energy for verbal processing.

"Okay, I don't have to talk. I was just going to ask you what position you want me in. Legs wide open?" He nods and opens the notebook.

The first pen marks go down scratchy. I look at his face and see his intense focus. Then I look away from his face. I look at his face, away from his face. I hear heavy shading from his pen. Broad, firm strokes. Then short, staccato lines.

In about two minutes he's done and hands the notebook to me, barely making eye contact. I look down at wild, black pen lines that indent the white page. A candle flame. An abstract desert woman with her arms raised in a V, dancing. My vulva. I've always admired the way Lloyd can summon frenetic lines into a form on the page.

What moves through me is a swirl of relief and peace. I'd told him that this exercise could help *him* learn my vulva, but I didn't realize how much I needed to see for myself. Alongside every vagina in a textbook, alongside every pinup pussy, I can now add this image. A page that was empty is now a page that is me.

"Don't ask me what that was like for me. I'm not ready to talk about it," he says.

I'm jostled from my peace, as if he's shut a door in my face. If I were going to say anything, it would have been *Thank you.* Now heat begins to swell under my skin like a bee sting.

"I'm not going to ask how that was for you," I say, tongue thick. I exhale and continue. "I do want you to know that the story I'm telling myself is that you think my genitals are disgusting, and you don't want to look at them. Because if I make you look, you will no longer be attracted to me."

I'm pushing the boundary line to keep talking. A couple years ago, I wouldn't have pushed, for fear of warping into the pushy men who've hurt me. But maybe I deserve to say my feelings, too, and knock on the door that Lloyd has closed. Maybe it doesn't make me a wicked woman, bloody sword in my hand. There are moment-to-moment births and deaths of intimacy. Sometimes it's hard to tell which way it will go.

We look into each other's eyes for a moment before I shift mine to the white shutters, layered shut like scales.

"Well, I don't know what story is true," he says, "but as it turns out, I'm still attracted to you. You're very brave. You're so wonderful . . . and I'd like to go to bed now."

We say *Good night*, but immediately, more words rustle between us in the silence. I'm not done. A couple months have passed since the last time when I asked him to look at my vagina, and he still has a similar level of discomfort. Has he even tried to unpack his feelings—in his journal, in his miles of running, in his therapy sessions? My thoughts rub into my pillow. Monologues begin to play out in my head like when I was a little girl buzzing in bed after my parents fought.

To me, this is making love, I will tell him tomorrow. This vulva drawing is making love. I know it's strange but this is where my love wants to go. Will you come with me? Are you willing to summon your courage? If I've bled every month for eighteen years so that my body could build our children, if I tore open to become a doorway for new life, if my genitals were sewn back together with a needle while I was awake, if I did the ninety Kegels a day, if I had my scars burned and my tissue killed, it doesn't feel like too much to ask you to look.

His body next to me feels prickly, and even the slight slant of the mattress on the bed feels like a part of him that I don't want to touch.

I've often heard that as a kid, all Lloyd needed to be content was a pencil and a long roll of unused newsprint. His editor dad brought home the end rolls. By high school Lloyd hatched his own secret art project of creating one-by-one-inch sketches of fuzzy cartoon characters he named *hair-balls*, which he deposited all around campus. His cheerful sketches were taped next to my side of the bed in Holly Springs. A hedgehog on a mountain trail with a speech bubble said, *Remember me, Cas, when your path is riddled with foxes.* A fox licked his lips in the distance.

My vagina has been chemically burned five times now. I need a witnessing of my tender center outside of the exam room. An equal and opposite force. I am determined not to fall into despair about my body, and an act of mutual creativity can keep me from sliding there.

This is the spirit with which I propose a project: thirty days of vulva portraits. I will sit and he will sketch for two minutes each day. Showing up to witness no matter if we're scared, exhausted, self-conscious. Because I have to be in this body every day whether he joins me here or not. And joining me here helps me feel his love.

"Sometimes I feel like I'm trying to channel the fun and the curious, but you receive something else. Something serious and intense," I say. "I could just be pushing the sexual part of our relationship to the side and ignoring it or shutting down. But I'm not. I hope you can appreciate that."

I tell him about the cultural conversations that have sprouted around *enthusiastic consent,* and how the enthusiastic piece often eludes me. But for the vulva drawings, I feel that big *yes.* Healing can mean following one yes to the next.

"I want to see you. I want to stare into you. I want to know you," he affirms. He stands up to gather the notebook and the pen.

VULVA PORTRAIT 4. "It's getting more comfortable and familiar . . . like a camp bunk bed," he says as he settles in by my feet. I laugh, despite visualizing the creak and leak-stains of camp beds. He's always had an odd angle for compliments. One time on date night, I was sitting on a patio in front of a distressed cement and brick wall and he asked to take a picture of me. The gray weave of my sweater matched the patchy background. *You look so good next to that wall,* he gushed. *It looks like you have concrete dust all over your shoulders, like you ran into a mixer truck.* Our eyes went prismatic with light because we knew our own private language would never let the world go stale. He saw me not as an object of allure in the foreground, beckoning, but as a natural figure of the environment.

In this one, he zooms in his perspective, drawing the layers of labia. There they are: majora and minora. Cosmic in proportion. So much clearer to me than the Big and Little Dipper in the sky, which I still struggle to find even though the sky's above me every night.

VULVA PORTRAIT 5. A change in his eyes. When he looks at my vulva, he looks with fluency, with invitation to explore. As an artist. He takes it in, fully, and I can see him observing and making choices. I feel the way I do when my doctor sits down on the stool and looks deeply in my eyes to listen, with no sense of urgency that she has anywhere else to be. As if this is the most important place. After he draws, he hands the notebook to me. My lips are more closed in this one, like a cowrie shell, and the lines sweep in coherent curves, as if they are collecting themselves. When I look at his sketch, I see coherence I didn't have access to before.

VULVA PORTRAIT 8. "You've got something there," he tells me casually as he stares into my vulva. I can imagine it: a foggy-white strand of secretion. My first response is a jolt of panic, which awakes from a younger part of me, before birth when he saw me poop on the floor, before pregnancy when he heard the phrase *mucus plug*, before my mid-twenties IBS and the hemorrhoid capsules that stunk like fish oil. I take a breath and land in this bed today, where it's okay to have a body with a vagina and a uterus that does uterine things.

"That's normal," I reply. "Right now I'm getting closer to ovulation, so my cervical fluid is getting stretchy and thick. Do you know why it does that? To be a good carrier for sperm." My ovulation fluid can get so voluminous that it actually reminds me of semen, I tell him.

"Whoa, that's really cool," he says. "I didn't know that. It does look kind of like semen." He begins to draw, both of us unafraid.

VULVA PORTRAIT 10. "What do you see as your first priority as a vulva portrait artist?" A news reporter voice issues from me. We've just watched a video clip of a new school board appointee.

"I have a huge learning curve here. I'm first responsible for just listening to *its* needs, not what I perceive to be its needs. My priority is to serve the vulva and to do what's best for the vulva."

"My mouth hurts. I'm not used to smiling this much," I say. We keep laughing, our mouths inches from each other. We embrace, and trade off between words and nuzzles.

"Draw this one with passion," I say. His eyes flare. This time he scoots off the edge of the bed to be at eye level with my vulva. A carefree and jubilant energy bats between us, something younger and freer. This is not an assignment. This is flirtation. This is foreplay. Actually, forget the *fore*—this is play, complete in itself.

At the end of the two minutes, I see that he's included more of my body. My thighs and the low curve of my belly appear for the first time. A new, integrated view.

VULVA PORTRAIT 11. As a girl I looked up the meaning of *Catherine* and learned that it meant *pure, virginal.* Being the Summer of Love teen I was, I felt chainmailed by this name. Years later I looked again, after I'd become an etymo-ho. I learned that *Catherine* comes from the Greek root *catharos,* the same root as *catharsis. The process of releasing strong emotions in a way that helps you understand those emotions.* The pure, it turns out, is a cleansing release, not a precious pearl of chastity.

This root changed everything. My name wasn't about what I held back, repressed, and clenched against. My name didn't center patriarchy and the threat of damaged goods. My name affirmed what I freely let flow from me, toward reckoning, toward peace. It was the first time my name felt as if it was my own, more yes than no.

VULVA PORTRAIT 12. "Which one is your favorite so far?" I ask.

"This one. This is the first one that turned me on the way you would expect a vulva to turn you on." I look down and see he is firm. "I want more of it. I want to stare into it, into the dark caverns . . ."

I'm already naked from the belly button down. Before he draws, I invite him to remove his pants too. He does, and our genitals do not demand full attention. They become one part of the body, stretched over words and gazes and soft kisses and laughter. His hardness, waving and tapping every now and then, is not a clockhand ticking toward penetration. It is communicating the same way his hands move through the air to tell an animated story. A conversation between our bodies.

"I like you here right now," I say. I push him onto his back, and we roll and tumble like cubs that might pull on an ear with a sharp tooth.

Both my hands enter the frame in this drawing, as if they're moving in closer to show him what's visible beyond the pen's capture.

VULVA PORTRAIT 13. Meredith, my sister-survivor, told me years earlier that J said he saw me at a restaurant wearing a lot of makeup and—*This is a lovely tidbit,* she warned—he said I looked like a whore. I have come to accept that in his mind I am a whore, eternally a whore. That whore lives and fucks and sings and lies and cheats. And that's the whore he wants.

Was I wearing the matte red lipstick? I wondered. The one I bought on spring break after I got the chin-length bob with bangs, when my mom and I said *coquette* and *gamine* all weekend, then I went back to school and a student said, *Look, there go Nicki Minaj.* I wracked my brain and realized I had never even stepped foot in the restaurant where he claimed he saw me.

Still, every now and then the phrase *somewhere a whore* blows into my mind, because part of me lives *somewhere a whore*, if only as a shadow puppet of J's hand.

I look away from how he looks at me.

VULVA PORTRAIT 16. I pass Lloyd the notebook, and he tells me he'll make this a one-minute sketch. A quickie. Rowan makes protest noises from the nursery, not quite crying, but I begin to get visions of him toppling over the edge of his crib. With each sound, emergency rooms and neck braces creep further into my mind. "Will you go check on him, please?" I ask. Pen in hand, Lloyd bounces half in our doorway and half in the baby's. "He's okay."

He continues to draw through the last thirty seconds as the grunts escalate next door. "I'll check on him again," he says. He puts his pen down and disappears. I think of what he asked me in the car recently, tired and frustrated. *Can't we ever just fuck?* I wished I could tell him *yes*. I hoped to someday tell him *yes*, that sex didn't always need to be elevated to some holy communion or a careful repair of torn fabric. But I said, *No, I really can't.* I had the urge to add *I'm sorry*, but I didn't.

"Are you all sucked out?" he calls from the next room. I lift my breasts to check if there's any milk left.

"Bring that baby here," I sigh, unstrapping my nightgown. Baby takes my flesh into his mouth so quickly it feels as if my milk rips a seam. I glance at the paper. My C-section scar stretches like a horizon line, and the shadow of my belly floats like passing storm clouds.

VULVA PORTRAIT 22. I'm walking the neighborhood when I realize that I think about my vagina more than I think about J now. Maybe every noticing of my vagina's sensations takes space that my memories used to fill. Something about physics, about *no two objects can occupy the same space at the same time.* J's voice and shape are getting edged out, replaced with my dough folds of humming, trickling, breathing. Yes, I feel my vagina breathing. Air moves through the lips. But it's about my imagination too. How I was hurt is becoming less interesting than my vagina's inhalations and exhalations. I don't know of a more right-fitted justice than this: a man took something from my body, and now my body replaces his image with its own.

VULVA PORTRAIT 25. "I know I keep saying *one more time*," Dr. S says about the silver nitrate after she burns the scars. "I'm hopeful the next time will be the last."

These scars, these kudzu scars, thrive even where they're uprooted.

End of June, twilight. I'm surprised to find purple flowers on the kudzu at the park where I stroll with Lloyd after our date. Kudzu has flowers? The blossoms are within view of the apartment where I lived with J.

I try to pull a flower off the vine, and it resists, with a fibrous connection. When it lets go at last, I hold its stalk. An arch bends like a long-haired, fluffy tail, something I want to stroke and pet. Yet it's solid and structural, expressing the stubbornness of the plant even as its softness invites me closer. I notice the upper flowers are actually quite pink when the light passes through. Turns out some colors can be seen only when four inches from your face, in the intimacy of your hand. I bring the flowers to my nose and there's a subtle fragrance that I can hardly detect—*grape syrup?*—and yet, when I set the flower down on the bench, I still smell grape when I inhale. That's the other thing about love: if you want to smell a flower, your brain fills in half the scent.

Even kudzu, the mile-a-minute invader, flowers.

Lloyd and I go home from our date, and he draws me. The ink he chooses: purple. Purple like a bruise. Purple like a flower.

arroyo

Our garden was a wonder in the dry land where you really had to commit to cultivating anything but dust. When we arrived in Santa Fe, our landlord, James, gave us a garden tour and a hand-drawn map of all the plants in the yard. We had dogwood, a peony tree, mugho pines, plum trees, butterfly bushes, roses, silver berry, trumpet vines, mountain mahogany, elm trees, crab trees, and silver lace. James would do most of the yardwork, although we were responsible for watering the plants in the front and keeping the silver lace, a flowering creeper, under control.

In the garden, I pulled up persistent elm shoots and spent time with the word *stress*. Who was I to be stressed now? I thought PTSD was for survivors of war zones, childhood abuse, and witnesses of horrific murder. But I'd found myself back at the ER again with heart palpitations, and a new cardiologist asked me, "Are you under a lot of stress?" Nothing greater than lifting thirty-five-pound bags of duck and pea dog food at my job at the veterinary hospital.

This year of Lloyd's graduate program was designed to feel like an extended vacation for me. I'd hoped that in the

Land of Enchantment, my heart could learn its true rhythm again, inside adobe and turquoise and big sky. We'd hike in slot canyons, revel in Georgia O'Keeffe's labial flowers, rate which restaurants had the best margaritas on the rocks. Very little was required of me, and that's exactly what I wanted after my two years of intense teaching. I walked dogs, emptied litter boxes, and handmade a cardboard E-collar for a pet rat recovering from surgery.

"Do you have any recommendations for me?" I asked the doctor, pen in my hand. I wanted to fix this heart problem, take up swimming laps, eat the right heart-healthy nuts.

He paused for a moment and smiled. "Live boldly. Do anything you want to do. Know that your heart poses no limits." He said it as if he wanted to break a one-mile chain that was attached to my ankle. Like releasing a dove to the sky. Like a provocation.

I'd spent so many hours sick in bed on a drip infusion of *Law and Order: SVU* in recent years. Why was I so devoted to those storylines, the search for answers of violently violated women, the search for justice? I still wanted to believe I had *moved on*, as if I'd jumped over some treacherous wall to all the good things on the other side, leaving the rest of it behind. I'd made it. I'd been away from J almost as long as I'd been with him. At this point it felt shameful when he popped into my head, as if I was hanging on to feelings for an ex-boyfriend while I'd loved Lloyd for three years.

My body was telling me: *Something has lodged itself under your flesh that is still with you.* Even after exchanging six thousand words with my hummingbird sister, the impact of the abuse was not clear. *Abuse* was still unnamed, shadowy in my arteries, in my bowels, in my sinus cavities. In every place where fluid moved, at the center of every passage, was an

obscure pain that lingered and baffled specialists in its origins. *Stress*, they continued to say with a furrow. *No medical
explanation.* I sought answers for a pain that was sometimes
a sharp and spastic fist in my abdomen, sometimes a dull
ache in the knot of my colon where it made a sudden turn.
Sometimes the pain hung onto my heart, dragging me as it
raced ahead. I was twenty-six years old, and my medical history was becoming a scroll. My marriage also wrinkled under
unnamed stress. Sex had not become something I desired
again, even after the stress of teaching was behind me.

One Thursday morning in November, I found a letter from
Lloyd on the kitchen table, with a flourish of his artistic cursive at the top: *My Darling.*

I am sad this morning, he wrote. *I feel like we have closed
off ourselves from the world of sex.* He went on to mention
a conversation from a few weeks back when I'd told him, *I
don't want you to feel like you're walking on eggshells.* The
thing is, after I said it, he realized it was a perfect description
for how he felt.

There's an us *link that needs to be mended,* he wrote, *something that brings us to an intimate stance.* He spoke of two
planets circling the same sun, sending out radio signals, every
now and then crossing each other's elliptical paths. To the
side, he drew an illustration of these planets and their orbits.

*I want to work on lovemaking, on sex, though I don't know
where to start after this writing. Well, yeah, I know I want to
lie naked touching each other for awhile, not taking each other's presence for granted.* His writing moved into the mar-
gins now, each thought connected by a separate arrow, one
making way for the next.

But that's not enough. I want us to talk about sex too. ~~~>
*Because we're just going through motions of obligation
every week or so . . .* ~~~>
and *I'm afraid it's me who is obligating you, which is why
I'm afraid to press you* ~~~>
Since I feel like it has something to do with J.

I have to turn the page to the side to read the last lines,
which curve around the binder holes.

*Cas, I'm sorry if any of this has made you uncomfortable,
but I've been uncomfortable for a long time, and I think you
have too. Thanks for listening. I love you. Your Husband, —L*

I didn't feel discomfort. Nor did I feel hurt. What alarmed
me was how I felt nothing. It didn't even feel as if the words
were written to me.

While he was out running the railyard trail, I wrote back to
him. *Dear Lloyd love.* I started with a blue pen, but one sentence in, the ink faded and broke, and I switched to black. I
told him the truth about my numbness, about my distance.
*I don't mean to be callous, darling. I'm just coming to terms
with the hard facts.* I said that I'd become self-centered and
hadn't been fighting for us, while also recognizing that in
other ways I'd been hard on myself and expected myself to
snap back more quickly from the intensity of teaching. *Tell
me how to fight for you because I feel like I've forgotten,* I said.

I didn't mention sex or J anywhere.

When he returned home, I gave him space to read. He
wrote me another letter, the third passed between us before
noon. *Dear cas.* This one included specific responses to my

question of how I could fight for him, and he named touches that would help him feel loved and connected. Simple things like turning toward him in bed and hugging him. Trying not to laugh as a default response to his touch. Whispering sexy things into his ear. Trying a new position.

This letter terrified me because nothing he asked for was extreme, and yet it still felt out of reach.

By winter 2013, four years after my escape, our desert garden was covered in snow. I bought a book called *The Sexual Healing Journey: A Guide for Survivors of Sexual Abuse*.

Maybe I could do this work only far from home, where my enchantment with the novelty of the desert could keep my past's swampland from swallowing me. Colors populated my vision that I'd never witnessed in nature. Gray-purple desert brush and orange mesas. I learned the word *arroyo*, a dried creek bed, because we walked our two dogs in an arroyo near our house. We lived on Oñate Place, and my mouth formed fresh shapes to curve around tildes and street names with *calle* and *camino*. I felt the touch of a new environment on my body, air light and crisp, not the hot, wet breath of the South. I woke so thirsty in the dry night that my throat felt wrapped in lizard skin, a thirst beyond thirst, the first gulps of water shaking down like sand. I cut off all my hair, sensing even my follicles craved new sensation.

I opened the sexual healing book not to understand my past but to understand what remained, like how to stop the disgust that surged when I glanced at the dark curve of Lloyd's body in bed before I reminded myself which man was here. I didn't want to reach toward the past; I wanted to reach toward the future. But the past still had blood that needed to be oxygenated. The past took a route through my heart.

Were you unable to give your full consent to the sexual activity?

yes

Did the sexual activity involve the betrayal of a trusted relationship?

yes

Was the sexual activity characterized by violence or control over your person?

yes

Did you feel abused?

yes

One *yes* could indicate sexual abuse. I put checkmarks next to all four. The abuse extended much further than the rape at the end. Emotional abuse. Verbal abuse. Sexual domination, manipulation, and exploitation. I had known this at a halfway level, but the truth came out of the background and into focus, as if before I could identify something only as *a tree* and now I could say *loblolly pine*.

I was abused. I was sexually abused. I was emotionally abused. I was restrained, held hostage, and terrorized.

While I read, Lloyd was in evening class, probably discussing Wittgenstein's conceptions of logic and language. I was coming face-to-face with the word *victim* for myself and *perpetrator* for J. As I took in the words of other victims and underlined phrases like *creative ways of coping*, I felt water beginning to rush through the arroyo of my memory. Up to my feet, up to my legs. What had felt like our own private struggle, our own private pain, now filled up subheadings and chapters. These were documented patterns and behaviors. *Victim.* I said the word aloud. One solitary word. *Victim.* So hard to pair the cold distance of that word with the rooms I shared with J where, over years, the word became mine. My favorite Wilco album playing. My glasses folded on the nightstand. The mouth that said *I love you.* The chin that tickled my clavicle. Pictures of us flashed in my mind, silly pictures with my underwear on J's head and us sitting on the floor at his gig holding each other's chins, our mouths comically open as if screaming on a roller coaster. Now the words *victim* and *perpetrator* were embossed over us like a watermark.

Sometimes I'd wondered, *Why'd you have to do it, J? Why'd you have to steal all our good memories, all our good songs? Why couldn't you have just been my first love, an ex-boy-friend?* But tonight, with this word *victim*, I had a hard time looking at any of the memories and calling them good. On every one of them, the letters swelled: V I C T I M.

I heard the door open. Lloyd walked in and stomped snow from his soles on the mat.

"Hello-beautiful-Cas-my-love." It came out of his mouth like one cursive word, warm. He smiled, cheeks ruddy from winter at high elevations, and in his hand was a paper plate with two slices of pizza. I put down my book. I opened my hand to receive food, my mouth to say *Thank you.*

February. A message from Meredith, my hummingbird sister, one year after our first conversation. *I don't want to be a ghost*

haunting you bringing up J. But remember I mentioned run-
ning into him? Well, we started talking again. I am embar-
rassed that I fell for this again.

My heart sank. I knew this cycle, kudzu roots spreading
even after the clearcut.

She was going to get away from him for good this time.
She'd been doing her own research to understand his behavior and how it ensnared her. In the space of a year, she'd
learned to say *abuse*, too, and I'd learned to say *trauma*. Five
thousand more words would pass between us over a week.

When I opened my laptop to type my next response to
Meredith, I could feel how fresh her anger and sadness were.
Words like *weak* and *stupid* swirled in her sense of self. I told
her: *Don't think you were stupid. We want to believe in love.*
We want to stand by people we love who are suffering. We want
to give second chances and give the benefit of the doubt. These
are good things. We just gave these things to the wrong person.

She grieved, *I think the only way to end things with him is*
for him to hate me. That way it's his choice. This reality also
shook me. I never wanted an enemy in the world, someone
who hated me, when all I wanted was to love well. His hatred
felt like the last word, and I couldn't make it right, which I
could see clearly now that Meredith grappled with her own
jagged ending. I guess that's why people say things like *For-*
giveness is for you.

Because his hatred of us doesn't get to be the last word.

There was a night when Lloyd and I were driving through the
desert, and our headlights lit up the small patch of road in front
of us. Everywhere else, darkness. A sparse, folksy song came
on, and the lyrics I knew filled the arroyo. Tears began streaming down my cheeks. I felt the four years that had passed since
escaping, a plume of peace about what I'd endured, and all that

had managed to grow in me since then. Tenderness for myself wrapped me like a weighted blanket because I had been abused, and yet here I was, in a car with my two dogs, my beloved, and my voice that was singing an old song with new feelings. As if to say: *My body went on and lived a whole lot despite what you did to it.*

Is this forgiveness? I wondered, surprised by the thought. How did forgiveness sneak into the car while I was processing my victimhood and my survival? But this wasn't the forgiveness that J's mom was asking me to grant in that voicemail years ago, a message delivered to help him feel better about himself in the wake of what he'd done, to help him move on. This wasn't the forgiveness I gave him over and over in order to end arguments without more harm done to my body and psyche. This wasn't connected to my young identity as a *forgiving person*, a big-hearted girlfriend trait. For years, forgiving meant ignoring my own needs to accommodate more space for J's pain while I made my own self smaller. No. This was something new. This forgiveness felt like my own self getting bigger, stronger.

This forgiveness could be felt only in full safety; my body was 1,043 miles away from the perpetrator, a distance that allowed me to stop bracing and to soften. The warm expansion of my belly moving with my breath, my lungs filling with air, and my voice singing. Still singing. Just like I did with him. Safe now, I could acknowledge that there *were* pieces of our relationship that made sense and *were* life-giving, and those pieces coexisted alongside the destructive ones. I could appreciate the complexity of my decisions and forgive myself for having fixed my eyes on the pieces of us that made sense as he spiraled into violence, for clinging to those pieces as the rest of our love disintegrated.

I could see the layers of who J was while also relaxing my need to understand the choices he made, graphing coordinates of how calculated versus how driven by mental illness. Forgiveness felt like accepting that there would never be any kind of reconciliation between us; I still existed *somewhere a whore* to him, and yet I needed to neither hate him nor forget the harm. I could hold the multitudes of who I am, who he was, who we were, and I loved that expansive quality of myself. It was both a part of what made me susceptible to his cycle of abuse and a part of what helped me to survive and heal. I was the one who was held hostage, coerced into filming a sex tape, threatened with Mace and raped, and yet I still had hope and love for the world? How did I get to be that fierce and beautiful? I pressed my palm over my tender, pulsing heart.

J's emails went to a hidden folder that Meredith said she never opened, just like the folders I had set up in my own account. But her messages? I read every single one. Over and over. And she did the same with mine, she said—*to keep reminding myself, to weed out what's real and what's brainwash*. We said, *I'm here for you*. We said, *I think you are incredible!* My hummingbird sister, she is iridescent. It is in her nature. When I see it in her, I can better see it in myself.

I didn't yet know that the peace of this forgiveness for myself wasn't a permanent state; I would cycle in and out of it as light hit my life at different angles and as new shades of the trauma were illuminated; the legacy of the violence kaleidoscoped. But forgiveness also felt like trusting myself to feel whatever I needed to feel next, to discern where my flares of sadness and anger wanted to go, toward what action, toward what justice, toward what healing.

The air was cool on my nipples and between my thighs. The sun smattered through the bamboo like ripples of light in irises. I was naked in this light, filter of the chlorophyll of spring. Here at the Japanese-style bath up the mountain in Santa Fe, Lloyd soaked on the co-ed side while I opted for the women's bath. Two women who looked like mother and daughter wore one-piece bathing suits, but I sat back in the chair with my uncovered skin rounded by the immensity of the sun. I thought of the mermaid-haired girl I was as a freshman in college, painted seafoam green and photographed nude. She was still here, naked and free. That brought me peace.

Also true was that she had changed amid the violence of abuse and in the years of coping as a survivor. Ideas I'd encountered in the sexual healing book seeded a whole landscape in my mind as I began to map the trauma's impact on my sense of self as a sexual being. I was beginning to understand why I didn't want sex, why desire felt so far away.

Healing felt like pushing a dark seed into the dirt to cover it in darkness, water it, and watch for the day when a shoot of green would rise above. The seeds I pushed into the dirt and covered with soil in patches of sunlight sounded like this:

I am limited in the types of sexual activity I feel comfortable with. I like it to go the same way. Always the same. I initiate. I can't be approached for sex without feeling cajoled, pressured, compromised. I want to be only on the bottom these days. Maybe because when I was with J, I could orgasm only on top. Oral sex now disgusts me. I want nothing in my mouth. I don't even like kissing.

Sex feels uncontrollable. Intellectually, I know that Lloyd doesn't want to hurt me and is a safe person. But sex feels like a wild force that divorces men from themselves, their goodness, their love. Sex feels impulsive and unpredictable. I worry about unleashing something in him that will hurt me, something insatiable.

I am a sexual object. "When we were at the party, you hardly looked at me while you're talking," I told Lloyd one night. "But then when we came home, you wanted to have sex. I know it's not true, but how I feel is that you don't want to talk to me; you only want to have sex with me."

During sex my mind feels separate from my body. "Cas, what are you doing?" Lloyd paused and asked me while he was inside me. I realized only then that my fingernails had been raking his back for bumps of blackheads, scratching capsules of oil to the surface.

My earlobe squished against Lloyd's skin, and I tried to take in his smell. Often I smelled him in opposites, absences. No cigarettes, no French fry oil. This meant I was safe. He was on his back, T-shirt off and jeans buckled. I inhaled. Fresh smell, peppermint castile soap. Neutral smell, skin that hasn't gotten sweaty since washed.

There would be no kissing, no touching with hands tonight. All we would do was listen to each other's heartbeats. I wanted a break from sex, weeks and maybe months when I knew he wouldn't ask me, and I wouldn't be waiting to be asked, and I wouldn't initiate eventually just because it seemed like time after my *noes* filled the arroyo.

"Please trust me," I said. "I'm not trying to move away from you; I'm trying to move closer. This is me trying to fight for us."

And he trusted me, even though a pause on sex wasn't what he would have chosen.

In the morning, the kids across the street bounced and jumped into the air, laughing as they rose above the adobe wall. I could hear the creaking of the springs, but I couldn't see the trampoline. I watched their small bodies levitate into wide-open sky.

REDEMPTION
OF THE PENIS

My breasts are long and flexible, emptying and filling like pitchers all day and night. When they empty, they hang long and soft. And when they fill with milk, they stand high and erect.

I lie on my side in bed and pull my baby closer to my breast. His mouth opens wide in anticipation. I squeeze my breast to guide between his lips, where he pulls me in. He gulps with little clicks, and that's when I know milk is flowing. And it hits me. Oh my. Since I was young, I've thought of the female body as a receiver, a place that accepts a penis, a vessel that holds a baby. But what am I doing here in this moment? I am sending my body into my baby's mouth. *He is receiving me.*

The next morning, I wake up milk-soaked with rock-hard breasts. Rowan has slept longer through the night, leaving me engorged, two wooden barrels of milk strapped to my chest. I've leaked warm fluid all over my shirt, and when I sit up, more milk tips out, so heavy that I have to cup one breast in each palm to the bathroom, where I express streams into the sink. My breast veins swell green and purple with totality.

They lied! I want to cry in a wondrous fury. *The whole culture lied!* A woman is not just a soft, enveloping home, and the vagina is not just a *sheath*, as the Latin origins suggest. I'm not only a receiver; I'm a born sender.

No one told me that I would enter a period of life when my breasts went hard, and I sprayed liquid to the walls, like wild hoses in spring. They didn't tell me that in pregnancy my belly would change from soft to erect over ten months with a pressing need of expulsion. A *bump*, they called it. My firm belly, rounded with blood and bone, would hang like a living sac between my legs in those final weeks. For hours in labor the bone-bulge would descend from my vagina as my pelvis canyoned.

"Do you think it's okay to have your own sexuality separate from your partner?" Kristen asked me before I got pregnant with Rowan. I had never considered my sexuality in those terms before, but once I did, I felt a new glimmer that rather than a response to male desire, my desire could be its own strong voice, its own declaration, its own question.

I am the mother of hardness. I know hardness as my own.

Sunday afternoon I run my fingers along Lloyd's skin while he lies still. Circles around his belly button, stripes up his chest, constellations connecting his freckles, spirals on his thighs. I touch with curiosity and innocence, skin of summer light.

"May I lay my head on different parts of your chest?" I ask.

I lean my head over his breastplate and hear his heartbeat. I lay my head between the crib of his ribs and turn my face toward the soft cavity of his belly. My ear on his stomach, I hear bubbly glubs. This is the body of the one I love, who once wrote to me, *Our love leaves cardboard fantasies to rot.* The one who has wiped my postpartum blood off the bathroom floor, the one who reads our children stories. Our sons. Someday they will be lovers. I hope they get touched tenderly, lovingly, respectfully. I hope their bodies are honored.

His penis stands directly in front of my eyes. I look at it with peace: *Do you think you and I could be friends? You don't look so scary. Tell me about yourself.* All this close looking at my vulva has made me realize that I've hardly studied his body up close in years. His skin wraps velvet-smooth like magnolia petals, taut around his slender frame. A meadow dips between his hipbones. Tiny pink areoles bud into shy nipples.

"May I touch your penis?" I ask. *Yes.*

I let my curiosity lead. My finger traces the contours as if reading his skin, letting a new story emerge. What if for awhile I could forget the history of penises? Could I let all of it fall away, a lifetime of associations—dick pics, impeachment, bukkake, titty fucking, wet dreams, blacklight crime scene splatter? Could I forget it all, the gallery of penis racket, all the blood flowing out of men's heads and into their dicks? Forget raping, coercing, colonizing, lying, entitled, territorial penises? Forget Zeus in all his inseminating forms?

The whole weight of the patriarchy has been held in his penis. So when he's next to me in bed, he's not just my lover but a throbbing piece of the patriarchy. Who wants to make love to the patriarchy? He's come to me engorged with #MeToo, the wage gap, and the defiled, pussy-grabbing office of the presidency. Before he has touched me, I first had to deflate his penis from all that poison.

What if I could see his penis as original innocence? Could I forget the other penises I've known and the ways I've touched them? Could I forget about the scripts of what a penis wants, the way my wrist learned to move in metronomic pleasing? What if I could touch it like his other skin, with gentle exploration and caress? Could I let his body just be his, loved?

I lamb my fingers along his lower belly, and goosebumps lift to meet my skin.

It's not the first time I've challenged my perception of the penis. In our childbirth class in my first pregnancy, each couple volunteered to research a topic. One of the topics: circumcision. I signed our names next to it.

"It's a personal choice," both my former gynecologist and our pediatrician said. The evidence of the benefits is not significant enough to recommend circumcision. The American Academy of Pediatrics backed this up: "The final decision should still be left to parents to make in the context of their religious, ethical and cultural beliefs."

Our insurance wouldn't cover circumcision; we learned it's considered an elective or cosmetic procedure.

Of the procedure itself, my former OBGYN explained: "The newborn physicians at our hospital don't actually cut off the foreskin. They use the Plastibell method. A bell-shaped piece of plastic is tied to the foreskin. Blood circulation to the foreskin is cut off, so the tissue dies. After four to seven days, the foreskin falls off with the bell."

Her tone suggested that this technique was gentler than the scalpel, but Lloyd's eyebrows arched as he asked, "So, the foreskin becomes necrotic tissue?"

"Yes, pretty much." The doctor let out a small laugh at his synthesis. How I loved his agitator and disruptor core. He wasn't afraid to explore an option for his son that diverged from the familiar form of his own body.

Among my friends, the circumcision decisions were split, and while I respected the nuances of their personal decisions, the conversations were even more clarifying for me.

"I don't want to have to ask my gross ten-year-old son if he's washed his penis," a friend joked of her decision to circumcise; both of us were pregnant with boys.

I realized right then that talking with my child regularly about his body was a priority of mine, with no shame or grossness attached to his genitals. An uncircumcised penis can accumulate smegma if not cleaned under the foreskin. But what's lost if we don't need to mention the regular care of a penis to our adolescents?

In my reading, I learned that the foreskin has more pleasure receptors than any other part of the penis. My first reaction? *Well, I've never known sex to be lacking pleasure for a man. I've been with only circumcised men, and they seemed to have plenty of pleasure, even more arousal than me, in fact. Why would a man need more pleasure than that?*

But once I was fully informed of the benefits and risks of circumcision, our consideration began to sound like: *Will we permanently remove part of our child's body after birth, with no medical necessity? Will we alter his genitals without his consent?* The answer was no.

Now that we've studied my vulva with the portraits, I find new curiosities. What does an adult's uncircumcised penis look like when erect? Flaccid?

I open my laptop for a Google image search, and my first impressions come from a deeply ingrained place. The uncircumcised penis looks indecent. I don't like it. It looks as if it's hiding something, a penis in disguise. Sloppy. I cringe that the word *animalistic* enters my mind, and I remember how Nana used to tell the story that when I was a little girl, I said of our brindle boxer, *Buster licks his peepee, then he licks my face.*

But then, as I get more acquainted, as I don't click out of the browser window to look away, my vision shifts. I see it: An uncircumcised penis has qualities that remind me of the vagina. I might even call it *layered, sheathed, mysterious.* It's made of outer and inner parts, and the unknown looms in the interplay of shaft and foreskin. The loose wrinkling of the foreskin reminds me of labia.

If I fear or have disgust at the appearance of the uncircumcised penis, that bias feels connected to a cultural disgust of the vulva. Ugly, dirty, holding smells. Suddenly the circumcised penis feels like a sanitized organ that's undergone a loss. We've taken away the intricacy of its construction, and I wonder how that has impacted our perceptions of the penis—and men—as one-dimensional, shallow, wanting only one thing.

A penis does not need to be a monument, a performance of confidence, a salutatory readiness. A penis can be shy, complex, layered. A penis can be vulnerable, ducking its head into its shell. A penis can retreat.

The darkened room, salt lamp glowing orange on my bedside table. I beam to Lloyd about my own hardness, how more things come out of my body than go in. Cyclical discharge, menstrual blood, milk. I tell him that when I seek the soft parts of his body and the hard parts of mine, edges of healing click into place for me.

"You know, the hardest penis is not necessarily the penis with the most pleasure," Lloyd reveals. My eyes go wide. I want more.

"The hardest penis is not necessarily the one that *gives* the most pleasure," I say, glowing. "I actually like it after you come, when you soften."

It feels as if we're telling secrets at a sleepover.

"I'm looking forward to decades of pleasure with you, with various levels of hardness," he says as he strokes my hair.

"Are you worried about your future penis?" I ask, knowing that advanced decades can bring erectile challenges.

"No. Because I have you."

Before we move our bodies closer, I sense the immensity of a careful labor ahead of us, as if we are building a cathedral together, and I don't know how I will muster the energy. He begins to rub my shoulders, back, and rump, deeply and slowly. He finds the places that ache from leaning my nipples over a crying mouth day and night. With one thumb over my shirt he rubs my nipple and exhales hot breath. Tingles spread roots like a milk letdown. Pleasure rings in me, and I remember. I release my bra, and he takes me in his mouth, softness melting into softness.

The baby sucks harder, I almost tell him, assurance that I can handle it. What he does to my nipples now I can barely feel, like a fly landing. He is surprised by how bottomless my body has become, tongue sent deeper into the well than the rope can reach.

I pull down my pants. He slides out of his.

Our genitals meet playfully, as if they have their own wagging tongues. They tumble, echoing softness and firmness and wetness and smoothness to each other. They curtsy and bow. They reach for each other in the dark. They remember every name. Until there is one name they can't remember, and that's when I guide his body on top of mine.

When he presses against my chest, my milk pushes out. Warmth trickles down each side of me, two tongues licking my skin.

We become long-muscled creatures beyond the masculine and the feminine. He feels more human than male, unified; I feel more human than female, unified. Loose-jointed, we rise beyond the forms of our bodies and our roles. Husband and wife. Mother and father. And yet, our bodies are not bypassed. Blood vessels and breath are close, swelling lips. We are full in our bodies, curving into each other, but how our bodies exist to the world doesn't matter. Here we are only ourselves. Here we are everything. We are sacred, stardust beings. We are ordinary beasts.

We surge together at the closest point, contracting.

Our one becomes two again. Our children sleep.

"It looks like an umbilical cord—still pulsing," he whispers, wonder of his own veined flesh in his hand. Yes, I was thinking of the moment of birth, too. He shone slick with me, the hair at the base of his shaft matted like the wet crown of our newborn's head.

cicadas

The sky held us like a tight womb, arches of pine and oak huddling us to the ground. Before living under the vast sky of New Mexico, I had never noticed how low Mississippi's ceiling felt, either oppressive or protective, depending on how you looked at it. Moving back home meant moving closer to the places where I had lived the saddest days of my life and where I had survived the scariest ones. But that's the thing about home. Home knows more of you than you would often choose to remember. Home is both sanctuary and haunting. If I looked at a map of this city, I would see a map of my own body. Where I ached, where I played, where I hungered and was fed. Where I opened, where I closed, where I opened again. I knew this city, and I chose it. This is the intimacy I moved toward.

We spent our first months in the suburbs at the Summertree House, the kind of tidy container couples inhabit when they prepare to reproduce. Streets were flocked with neon safety turtles tall as first graders, holding flags that cautioned, SLOW. But inside, the Summertree House still felt like death. Even the windows discouraged light, squeezing out sunlight at midday in a kaleidoscope of shadows. The light twisted, and I saw myself emptying commodes of my grandmother's hard-formed poop. Twist again, and I brushed hair that shed from her scalp in long, snakeskin sweeps.

We wanted to start a family soon. I couldn't welcome new life here. Mortality festered. This house was for endings, for the disintegration of bones from death-driving cells. In the cul-de-sac, I smelled whiffs of death, too, our neighbors smiling and waving from identical plots of lawn. On the faces of the houses, I saw the pallor of white flight.

LloydandIfellinlovewithaJacksonbackyardbeforeahouse, peeking over the fence to see a park-like plot of hundred-foot pines and mature oaks. A corridor of Japanese magnolias and bushy nooks for hide-and-seek. Our own secret garden in the city. In our new home, it wasn't uncommon to hear caravans of sirens and small explosions in the night, with some neighbors rushing to the private Facebook page to ask, *Fireworks or gunshots???* Backpacked people experiencing homelessness stood at the intersection a block away with signs saying, *HUNGRY.* A nearby gas station leaked brown paper bags of tallboys.

Did I feel less safe than in Summertree? Yes, I guess you could say that I did; I walked to my door with my house key between my fingers. But did it feel more like home? Yes. This place was our own, alive. Nesting didn't just mean curating a beautiful nursery and organizing the pantry. Nesting was not just for me and mine. It meant probing, *Which county and school district will receive our tax dollars? What will our children learn from the diversity of their classmates and teachers? Which systems will our life support?*

We're building a nest, but what's our nest building?

Half-Price Pint Night, the sun setting over the Whole Foods parking lot. I was sitting at a window table with four friends and Lloyd. Midway through my beer, I sensed a person walking past my shoulder. Once he passed, I saw him: the slow glide of his gait, the turnout of his feet, the tilt of his T-shirt across his shoulders, the curve of his elbow. It had been six years, but I still knew every piece.

Green apron strings were tied behind his back, so he must have been working. I knew he'd worked here in the past, but I was tired of keeping a map in my head of places to avoid and slinking around the city like prey. I'd turned down invitations to meet up here before, saying things like, *Oh, my ex-boyfriend might work there. He may be unsafe.* But this time I said *yes*. Why should I be the one who couldn't go _____ and do _____ while he had an all-access pass to anywhere he wanted?

And there he was. J turned around and saw me, interrupted movement in the swivel of his head. I pretended not to see him, training my eyes on a friend, while my peripheral vision tracked his motion. I became conscious that I was drinking a beer, like on the night that he raped me. *Always the same shit with you, Cathy*, I could imagine him saying. Should I leave? I took stock. We were not alone. I sat with five other people. Safety in numbers.

I looked at Lloyd as he spoke. His body emanated energy like a monk's, with a deep openness, along with a scholar's gusto during a philosophical disagreement. Lloyd didn't command the wall of macho protection that I felt next to my dad, my brother, and even with J, whose first impression was shy and kind. In Lloyd there was no impenetrable gristle of testosterone, force field of intimidation, or buzz of fight. The thing is, I liked the feeling of being protected, and sometimes I missed it. But I understood that whatever masculine rope of violence did not coil in Lloyd was part of why I loved him and why he loved me in a way that made me feel free. What felt like protection one day could feel like possession on another.

J sat down on a barstool by the window on the other side of the café. Perhaps he was on a break. But he didn't face the window. Instead, he turned his body to face mine. I kept my eyes on everything but him. But from the edge of my vision, I saw him raise his phone in front of his body and point the camera in my direction. Was he taking pictures of me? I nodded along to what my friend was saying, incomprehensibly. J's phone was still aimed at me, his arm fixed. Was he making a video of me? He began to laugh. Maybe I was being paranoid. Maybe he was just watching a funny video. But, no, he had his body turned unnaturally in my direction. A devilish laugh.

I considered telling Lloyd, who hadn't noticed J nor the shift in my energy.

I didn't want a scene. I didn't want a fight. I just wanted this to end. I froze, continuing to nod along to the conversation and tucking my hair behind my ear.

J sat on the stool for a few minutes and eventually stood up. He walked past me again, and I held my breath, our bodies only a couple feet from each other.

I couldn't take another sip of my beer. As soon as Lloyd finished his, I said I was ready to go. When we stepped outside, I hung onto his arm. "Move fast. Stay aware," I said. "J was in there."

Although startled into confusion, Lloyd moved into a more alert mode, his eyes scanning the parking lot as his back straightened. He opened the passenger door for me.

Once we were safely driving, I told him what had happened and my suspicion that J was filming me. Lloyd blinked and I watched his swallow stumble down his throat as he processed his totally separate experience, how he laughed with our friends while I sat in fear.

"Why didn't you tell me? I want to know these things. I need to know these things," he said. Not a voice of criticism but one of care, as if to say, *You don't have to endure this alone. I want to be there for you.* The trauma told me it was safest to endure it alone, though. I was the one with the practice of de-escalating J's power flares. We were most likely to get out safely if I managed it.

As Lloyd drove us home, I kept glancing in the rearview mirror to see if J was following us. My teeth chattered, and I wished I didn't know how vulnerable my body still felt in proximity to him. I wished I didn't know that he could still isolate me in a room full of people, even while sitting across from my husband. I had now been away from J longer than I had been in relationship with him, but this fear felt as raw as it had six years ago.

I decided to schedule a meeting to tell my principal about the potential threat of J. I was teaching again, and I'd gone through enough active shooter drills and lockdowns to be cautious. I'd never known J to own a gun, and he had a tenderness toward children, but I felt responsible for reporting any possible threat. Would he come to the school looking for me? He could easily find my workplace. My name, photo, and position were on the website.

When I sat in my principal's office, a wave of unexpected shame rose in my cheeks as I explained the shorthand of the truth: "I had an ex-boyfriend who stalked me in the past. He has a violent history, and I have current concerns for safety or that he may come looking for me." He asked for a picture to give campus security, and it felt like a replay of 2009. In some ways, it felt more humiliating because my professional identity now took on this watermark of victim. I wasn't just the fourth-grade writing teacher who sat in a circle on the rug with her students, composition notebooks open in front of us. I was also someone with a violent ex-boyfriend, with a past stalker, which felt like a red flag about my stability and judge of character.

Even if J wasn't a danger to me anymore, even if he wasn't filming me that day, I was angry that six years had passed and it was still necessary to have this conversation. I didn't yet know the term *intimate terrorism*, which I would learn from Rachel Louise Snyder's book *No Visible Bruises*. But our active shooter training taught us to look for and to report any warning signs that someone may be on a path to violence. Erratic, unsafe, or aggressive behaviors. Hostile feelings of injustice or perceived wrongdoing. I connected those tips to what I'd experienced with J.

There were many questions I'd asked over those years. One line of questions that persisted like kudzu: *Was it love? Can I really call it love, knowing what I know now? Or was our relationship better classified as hatred?*

"Gender hatred. The hatred against the independence and freedom of women." This is how author Cristina Rivera Garza characterizes the murder of her sister by an ex-boyfriend in her book *Liliana's Invincible Summer*.

Could the love and the violence be separated? Or did the violence bleed into every part of our history together? Could I pinpoint a moment when love morphed into hatred? Or was it there from the very beginning, a quiet predation I couldn't detect?

The thing about being a survivor is that at every stage of life you have new wisdom and perspective that's in conversation with the events of the past. I had two feet in adulthood: spouse, homeowner, dog mom, guardian of my students. Thankfully, I had an accumulation of healthy relationships with love and mutually respectful care. All of this made me look back on the relationship with an adult's eyes.

The day I had turned twenty-four, I was still teaching sixth grade in Byhalia, with the high school in view from where I parked my car. I couldn't hear my new age without thinking, *This is how old I was when we started dating.* I imagined what it would be like to date a seventeen-year-old. We would talk on the phone, and they might mention their homework, their parents, their curfew. I would have sex with a high school student, and maybe it would be that child's first sexual experience. Considering I was a teacher, this was deeply disturbing, illegal. I pushed it out of my mind.

After I began using the word *abuse*, I looked again. I searched for the definition of statutory rape and the age of consent in Mississippi. Sixteen. That's the age I was during our first summer of driving around Jackson listening to music and falling in love, before I turned seventeen on August 20.

And even later, I began to wonder: If I were in my twenties, what would attract me to a sixteen-year-old who had no life experience as an independent? That teenager would be accustomed to living under a parent's rules and making decisions within someone else's terms. Coming straight from childhood, they wouldn't know what life felt like without an authority figure. A boyfriend's control would feel similar, linked to love.

It became harder not to see J as a predator, even if his choice to date a minor came more from a lack of self-awareness, emotional immaturity, and deficits of self-confidence. Dangerous qualities for a man.

But there were still confusing crossovers and gray areas. One of my best friends had started dating J's bandmate at the same ages, connected through me, and they got married one month earlier than Lloyd and I. I was maid of honor in their wedding, and she was matron of honor in ours. They were still happy, and it was a relationship I respected.

To look again and again. That is the legacy.

A rhythmic whirring spun me when I stepped outside our front door. The air draped like a hood of humidity, and the drone of weed trimmers spun metallic in the distance. But this other sound was new. Loud and pulsing, like the buzz of high-voltage electrical wires. Even from inside the house, the hum called me like a distant siren's song. I couldn't unhear it.

"What *is* that?" I asked Lloyd. It prodded me, wouldn't leave me alone. A few days of the relentless humming passed before we hopped in the car to seek the source. We rolled our windows down, and I craned my neck out the passenger side to track the spiraling thrum. We followed the distant murmur, with me directing Lloyd to make left turns and rights until we dead-ended. In front of us electrical towers rose above the veil of kudzu swallowing pines.

I didn't feel we were at the exact center of the sound, but it was the only answer we could find for the phenomenon. We turned around and drove home.

The next day I saw the headline in our daily newspaper: *13-year cicadas emerge, ready for love.* I laughed out loud. The hum sounded so man-made, voltaic. Could it be? Insects were having a raucous summer of love. Male cicadas were singing mating calls all around us, gathered in trees known as *chorus trees* as they tried to draw interested females.

For thirteen years the cicadas had lived underground, larval nymphs sucking the fluid out of tree roots. Then all at once, they emerged from the ground, and for a few weeks, they would live in the trees as a brood of adults, devoted entirely to reproduction. Once the eggs were laid, the thirteen-year cycle of a new generation would begin. The nymphs would drop from the trees and burrow into the ground for more than a decade.

The summer of the cicadas, Lloyd and I became devoted to reproduction, too. *Have sex every other day from days ten to fourteen of your cycle*, my doctor prescribed. In our queen-sized, memory foam bed, we began the cyclical dance of conception.

Tuesday night sex. Before work sex. Yawny sex. Romantic date-night sex. Skip-the-foreplay sex. Distracted sex. Long and sweaty sex. The most sex we'd had in years. Sometimes I gasped quietly in orgasm. Other times I said, *You go ahead*, and I squeezed his ass cheek as if prompting a horse to gallop to the finish line while I reined him closer. My orgasm wasn't required. His was crucial, the orgasm that would produce babies. All I needed was the quiet release of an egg in my body, which I could neither sense nor control. I tried to relax into passion, but mostly I saddled into a strategic meeting of penis and vagina, the mechanics of bodies squishing, grinding, sliding.

Three months into *trying*, Lloyd walked to the bathroom, his male baton still jutting in front of him like a caricature of an erection. I lay naked on the bed, praying the sperm would land. I inhaled deeply, and I felt an empty square drop in my chest, sadness bordered with loneliness. A feeling with no color, an empty cellophane wrapper.

Hadn't I vowed to never find myself here again, having sex when my body didn't want sex but I said *yes* for other reasons? I could sense the accumulation of the *trying* in my body, three months of litter, so many empty cellophane wrappers discarded inside me. No baby, just more and more empty space. This can't be where our baby comes from, not this emptiness, not this finish line.

When Lloyd returned from the bathroom, I told him, "I can't keep doing this."

He scooted under the covers and wrapped his arms around me, his front soft and warm against my skin.

By September, the cicadas stopped their mating calls and burrowed back into the dirt. One night our bodies made a warm color in bed, joined in effortless rhythm after a festival of Irish dancing. The bowstrings of jigs, reels, and ballads still vibrated my eardrums.

The next month, I saw no blood.

Pregnancy hit me like a second puberty. Curious and enthralled, I became a newcomer to my own flesh. Like my adolescent days alone in front of the mirror figuring out what was what, I mashed and pulled on my skin, traced new curves, and finger-walked my breasts. My belly grew from bump, to mound, to bluff, to broad crag, each iteration thrilling and new. I imagined who I would become by the end of the process.

As my body changed into new motherhood, Mom's and Nana's bodies flashed in my mind as prophets. Mom's nipples were like radio dials. When, as a young woman, I watched her fasten her bra, the chunky knobs of her nipples enthralled me. I didn't understand how they could be so firm and assertive when mine were such malleable, shy cones. Sometimes I pinched mine to see if I could have that same shape of power. Nana's belly, a swinging escarpment, had a long, vertical scar that joined her at the middle from Mom's cesarean birth. Her breasts were broad sacks that smelled like French perfume, and when she placed a warm baguette in front of me on the table with rounds of Camembert, life felt yielding and whole.

PROUD FLESH

July is so hot that if you water your plants during the heat of the day, you risk burning the leaves under wet beads of sun. Still, the mosquitoes keep being born. I take a walk around the yard after the rain to turn over each nursery: the plastic sandbox, the empty pots, and the mud kitchen spoons. Maybe our story-founts are like this too. Filling and emptying. Filling and emptying. Pain here, pleasure there. And we'd never stop the rain because then it wouldn't all be so green and alive.

I return for my eighth meeting with silver nitrate.

"I'm not sure what's happening, but I feel burning in my rectum," I tell Dr. S as the silver nitrate seeps in. Her forehead wrinkles, and she peers deeper.

"Do you mind if I do a rectal exam?" she asks. I tell her to go ahead. She squeezes lubricating gel, and inserts one finger into my anus, one into my vagina. I feel her fingers meet and rub, my skin a thin rubber balloon between them. "It's closed," she confirms, eyes tilted to the ceiling. "My fingers are not touching. But your perineal body is extremely thin."

There's no muscle connected there, she finds. Only skin, where normally the perineal body is a confluence of muscle attachments.

Again, the question: *What happened here? Why?* A smear of heat spreads across my forehead and cheeks, the fear of something gone wrong in my midwife's repair. Maybe the muscles weren't reattached after I tore, Dr. S says, but it's also possible that my repaired muscles retracted on their own. Bodies respond to healing in different ways.

I'm not interested in probing if I was injured, not today. I may never know the answers to these questions. Still, the extent of the trauma is a persistent revelation.

Dr. S gives me a new word to add to my healing collection: *innervation.* It's the nerve supply of a specific part of the body. She explains that the nerves are so close between my vagina and rectum, especially with no muscle between them, that my brain can't yet perceive the difference. Since my genital structure changed and the nerves are regenerating, my brain is still making connections between the tissue and the sensations.

I nod along as I'm processing. There's been an emotional innervation for years in my body, wires crossed between danger and safety, violation and consent. Existing too close to each other.

My mind wanders to the skin bridge, to the way I like my ass tapped now, and I wonder if innervation has made new pleasurable routes of perception in the nerves. I let my thoughts rest on that rich possibility for a moment before my mind pendulates back to my vanishing muscles and my doctor's voice. *A potential genital reconstruction as you age* and *It's even more important for you to maintain your Kegels.*

This reality doesn't plunder me like the early sessions when my scar tissue was discovered. Maybe because I no longer believe I should have a body that doesn't require my daily devotion and my continual discovery. That sounds like both privilege and a lie now, born from a myth of bodily perfection, for a world built for productivity, where bodies function like machines. I hear the voice of the oppressor, insisting on sameness, where difference is threatening.

In my seeking, I've found dynamic bodily company in so many places. I've watched trans friends meet themselves in their gender-affirmed bodies for the first time, and I've watched a trans teen I know move out of state after hormones were made illegal for minors. I've watched friends with disabilities navigate bodies that look or move differently than most. I've watched friends go through fertility treatments, ruptured uterine cysts, liver transplants, bipolar disorder, autoimmune disorders. Lloyd told me the other day that he's had a twinge in his shoulder ever since Guider was born because of the way he rocked him in one precise armhold as he was falling asleep, night after night. I like knowing that fatherhood has left an imprint on his tissues, too, even a small one.

The body is not stasis, unchanging. There are imprints. Life has touched this body; lovers have touched this body; parents and genetics have touched this body; babies have passed through this body. Politics and legislation touch bodies. I have touched this body, and I know its scars and sensations. There's a lot I still don't know, but I do know that I'll show up for whatever questions I need to ask and seek support for what I find.

I'll return in a month to see if the scar tissue is gone. This may be my last treatment.

Mom texts me and says that Nana is threatening to take all her pills again. They're living down the street from us in a condo now, where Mom cares for Nana as she descends into dementia. Mom sends me messages of spare losses daily as they arrive, as Nana's memory departs.

"She can't remember Woodstock."

"She can't remember Notre Dame."

"Today she asked, 'Who's Antoine?'" My grandfather's name.

She complains of itching all over her scalp, as if each story departs her brain with a fizz, and she sometimes pulls words by the shirt collar to say, "Someone please shoot me." I don't bring the kids there past sunset because she has no filter when the episodes of desperation set in.

I drive over to help, less than a mile of silence between my babies and my matriarchs. I walk in to the tones of what could be a teenager arguing with her mother, as if they've stepped back in time. The voices have swelled into hours, rubbed raw. Their faces are raw.

"No more talking. We're done talking tonight," I declare calmly. Mom looks at me confused, but I repeat, "No more talking."

I hug Nana, and she starts crying into my shirt. I hold her shoulders and feel her give in. I pull a vial of lavender oil from my pocket and rub a drop on her wrist and one on her heart. I walk to my mom and do the same. The room is silent. I insist.

"Sit down." I lead Nana to the armchair. I stand behind her chair and begin combing my fingers through her hair. She closes her eyes. I move to her feet, skin cracked and white. She flinches when I touch a bruise on her shin, and I place two fingers as light as a kiss.

In the last year she's been saying, "When I die, don't say I was a cook." I hear her desire to be known for more than how she served us with her labor in the kitchen. At the same time, her hands prepared food that located me. Fresh mint and cucumber with lemon juice in her couscous salad. Onions, tomato, and turmeric in her paella, bursting with mussels and shrimp tails. Quiche Lorraine with shredded Swiss, jambon, and poivre. The earthy caramel syrup of her flan. The flavors she fed me were more than ingredients; they budded my tongue with knowledge of who we are. First, the tastes. Then, many years later, I found the words *multi-ethnic* and *multiracial*.

She can't show her love and heritage with food anymore. The other night Mom walked in and saw Nana setting chicken on the open burner with no pan, wrapped in plastic and yellow Styrofoam.

Kneeling in front of her now, I make the sign of the cross with my thumb on her forehead and say, *Hail Mary, full of grace*, knowing this will still mean something to her. I watch slow tears roll from her half-closed lids, elevators that give up their weight and sink to the floor, where her doors open to me. She opens her eyes and looks up at me. How does she look up at me when I am below her? I don't know, but she does. I cradle my hands on either side of her face, and I look into her red-veined eyes. Her skin under my fingers is tough, the wrinkles palpable seals over sun and grief and physical pain. How long has it been since someone really touched her?

"You're a miracle," she tells me. "Ever since you were a little girl, you always cared. You were always my miracle girl." I take in the guardian angel pendants that surround her, the Eiffel Towers, the gold crucifix on her chest.

For years I was recovering from giving too much. I had to learn a new way. But tonight I let myself be the miracle again. As I drive home in the dark, tears puddle at the edge of my ducts. I want to cry, but the waters stay right there at the edge, where I've learned to keep them. I hope that changes someday. I hope the tears will flow freely. For now, I dab my finger in the wetness in the corner, kiss it, and press it to the center of my forehead.

I'm back in the bathtub for soothing the nub of my scars. I find my fingers typing *hypergranulation* in Google again. It's like running my finger across prayer beads, a ritual now, connecting the reality of my body to some vast web of knowledge and nature. I click my way through articles and find these words: *proud flesh.* The term is often used to describe the granulation tissue that is common on horses' legs and hooves, the same scars I have. There's even a medi-cal definition: *exuberant granulation tissue in a poorly healed wound, characterized by florid, "geographic" scarring on the skin surface.*

Suddenly it feels like a brilliance the way my wound has worked overtime toward healing, creating a garden of tissue around the tear. *Exuberant. Florid.* Those are my vagina's words. *Proud flesh.* As if my body wanted to sing its own per-spective from the wound. What has been concealed will grow barbs and flower. Tenderest act of survival.

They burned my vagina once, twice, three times, four. They burned my vagina five times, six times, seven times, eight. My hands make ripples across the bathwater while the lines play in my head like a nursery rhyme. But the words *proud flesh* also begin to rise in me. They keep rising in me as

I towel myself off, as I soap the dishes, as I sit on the toilet, and as I push the stroller down my street the next day. *Proud flesh.* It sounds like a riot. Or a benediction.

Lloyd straps Rowan into the carrier on his body and we head toward a small clearing in a chain-link fence. Guider holds my hand as we walk toward a wall of dense green.

Beyond the trees and the fence sprawls a scaled hydraulic model of the Mississippi River, where concrete ruins snake across two hundred acres. The river basin model, built from 1943 to 1966, simulated water patterns, weather, and floods. Previously the Army Corps of Engineers had addressed flood measures along the Mississippi through localized, single sites, building locks, runoff channels, and levees. But this model was built to understand the entire river system, its tributaries, cliffs, lakes, plains, and levees all the way to the Gulf of Mexico.

"I remember the first time you brought me here," Lloyd says. He speaks of the magic when I parted the branches like curtains and told him to follow. The overgrown vegetation makes the basin model easy to miss. No signage. When we stepped into the clearing, he took in the secret world whose borders he'd run for years in cross-country meets. For miles and miles he had raced alongside this mystery.

"Oh wow, I forgot that I showed you this place first," I said. "I was thinking you showed it to me."

Now I don't know how I first came to this wonder. Did J bring me here? Did we ever come here together? It seems like a place he would have known. I search my memory as I scan for poison ivy while we walk, but nothing emerges. If J did introduce this spot to me, the memory is so thin that it's transparent, smoothed across the geography. I don't ask it to return.

I know only that for years I've come to this concrete contour of river, and today I bring my family. Guider lets go of my hand to jump along the banks, a new playground.

The late-afternoon sun twists through the trees and over the dry river's sinews, across the derelict slabs of concrete and weeds. If you didn't know this place, you might not call it beautiful. But this land opens into me, a dilation and effacement of so many iterations of myself that they blur together now. As in a stop-motion flip-book, I change almost imperceptibly from page to page, limbs and expressions and the swirl of my hair; but assembled in the quick flip of memory, I am running, I am running through this land. Through my first period, through my parents' divorce, through high school dances, through J, through falling in love again, through teaching, through birthing and birthday candles, through healing.

Can there be land more beautiful than the land that has grown me? Can a body be more whole than the one that is my breathing home?

As we drive out of the park, I find the letters *BARREN WOMB* spray-painted in brown on the side of a rusted barn. Friendly, with a wavy line, the words appear to be waving at me to join a party rather than a curse. In my imagination, I add sunflowers. Maybe a group of teens with uteruses have formed a punk band called *BARREN WOMB,* raging against the lawmakers who would protect their womb only when it's fruitful, multiplying. I'd have joined them in high school, hair to my waist and shaking a tambourine in the corner, wingtipped eyes.

I had a dream this summer that my first boyfriend was a teenager like me. His body was not ahead of mine; he was narrow and golden, hairs new and soft. Our hands learned a language together while my nana scooped seeds of a halved cantaloupe into a metal bowl in the kitchen. In this dream, we were naked but not nervous, and every time we touched, our skin was daylight and the room was big, with windows even bigger. Can you hear it, the origin story where no one wants to harvest grain between your hipbones? I awoke from the dream with my past warmed under sunlight. As if I grew from this green.

Healing grows in all directions, back to seeds, lush depths of soil.

I've often taken a pain tour of my past, touching the places that hurt and listening for the echoes of what can still be learned. But today I take a pleasure tour because that sound was also there, making me.

I was the little girl who made my great-grandmother Marie laugh when she visited us in Florida. We didn't speak the same language; she spoke only French and Spanish, some Arabic. But Nana says I kept her on the dance floor on New Year's Eve and didn't want to let her hands go. She laughed so hard she almost peed through her pantyhose.

I was the young woman camping with Mom, Nana, and Nana's boyfriend on a beach in Mexico. Mom and I took a nap on towels and when we awoke, Mom said sleepily, *Who are those naked people in the water?* I shaded my eyes to see it was my grandmother and her boyfriend, splashing like kids.

I was the one whose naked body was painted seafoam green and photographed like a mermaid, hair inky and fluttering, chest cresting over waves even as love hurled itself at me, netted around my ankles.

I was the bachelorette on the night my friends and I danced naked around a fire in the woods, shedding our dresses into the grass and freeing ourselves from clasps of elastic. The fire blurred our faces across the circle in summer moonlight. Our fire was whole; our fire was many separate flames.

I can see the brilliance of my pleasure, the brilliance of my body's survival through it all.

It's an August day, bright as the day I was born, when I sweat to the clinic to see if my hungry scars have left me.

"Looking good. The hypergranulation hasn't come back," Dr. S says, peering inside for one last time. I bring my legs back together and get dressed.

The ending is quiet, with no bell to ring or cake to cut. Oddly truncated, even though the postpartum visits lasted longer than we ever expected.

Ten months after my baby was born, my wound is healed.

I walk to the checkout desk, and for the first time in almost two years, there is no follow-up appointment to schedule.

We call it a *meander map*. The changing course of the Mississippi River has been mapped to reimagine thousands of years of its life, through erosions and floods and new corridors. The river is nimble, adapting to deforestation and alterations to the land. The cartographer and geologist Harold Fisk studied the river's movement, collecting twirling, divergent paths into one image. Like a subway map, distinct colors chart the river's courses across history. Looping and bending, the river crisscrosses and unfurls in shades of turmeric, salmon, fennel, egg blue, and apricot.

And I hear it: Healing is a force that meanders.

In the river, I see the alterations in the structure of my genitals, the twists and turns of sutured flesh, the loosening of ligaments from floating two big babies. New incarnations. The river responds creatively to changes in the land—messily. I do too.

August morning. Week of my thirty-second birthday. I wipe and instead of the gray slime of the past months, I find bright red blood. I wipe again, even more blood. I wipe again, and the blood streaks stronger, fresh-fruiting cerise. *Yes. It's back.* I knew that my menstrual cycle wouldn't return until my vagina was healed. My arms tingle that I was right, follicles alive with intuition. I've been waiting for this, the shed cycle that's not the death slough of silver nitrate.

When Lloyd comes home, I tell him the news. "Ah! Your cycle has returned!" He hugs me around Rowan, who's in my arms. Guider runs up amid the excitement, and in that moment, I know: my boys will learn about my menstrual cycle and a woman's biological rhythms. My blood will not be a secret whispered in the hallway.

I dream of a world where little boys have seen their mothers' monthly blood. I dream of an original knowledge of blood that is not violence but the power of creation from a womb. Not war or genocide, not video game combat, not school shootings, not concert shootings, not grocery store shootings, not nightclub shootings, not police shootings.

First, this blood.

By day three of my period, Guider enters my bathroom and sees me wiping blood. Heavy flow, dark fruits. He doesn't look worried because he knows this blood is normal, Mama isn't hurt. He is three and already he knows.

What do we call the blood that is our mothers'? You and me, breathing.

A vagina is more than a forgiving place. It is a bold organ of expression. A world-delivering place. A site of rebellious healing and defiance. It's powerful enough to mold skull plates. It cradles us all before our first cry. It's a celebration of regeneration, life continuing.

Soon after my blood returns, on the changing table, Rowan discovers his penis for the first time. His pudgy fingers stretch it like taffy. A sparkle of curiosity in his eyes turns to bubble-eyed wonder as he tests his organ's squishiness and begins kicking with joy.

"Did you find your penis?" I ask sweetly. "Rowan, that's your penis." He squeezes it, pulls, and hangs on as if he found the hand of a friend. Six tiny teeth gleam from his open mouth.

"Hey, guys, Rowan found his penis!," I call. Guider's reading a bedtime story with Lloyd in the room next door.

"Oh, wow! Rowan found his penis!" Lloyd calls back.

"Rowan found his penis!" Guider repeats with a giggle of glee.

In a moment, all three of us stand at the changing table celebrating Rowan's bodily discovery. He will not remember this day. He will not remember how we stood around him as if at an altar table, clapping and smiling, but I hope both my sons will grow into a wholehearted awareness of bodies as bodies, each part radiant.

I don't think I could have seeded this joy in the next generation without meeting the exuberance of my own body, all those hours learning my new genital shape in the bathtub and checking on my vulva's healing with the hand mirror. Without Lloyd holding space and witnessing in the vulva portraits.

The less I think about *raising boys* categorically and the more I think about raising Guider and Rowan specifically, two individual beings with their own needs and wondrous emergence, the more capable I feel, the less afraid. I will not be able to control their bodies, neither what they receive nor the choices they make. But as parents, we will teach them each day to be aware of their own bodies and feelings and to make respectful choices with others'.

And we won't do it alone. We will cultivate a community around us bent toward liberation. We will learn alongside each other, companion plants flowering with the same pollinating bees.

I will receive a text from a dear friend that my five-year-old didn't listen to her daughter's *Stops* in the backyard on the trampoline; and standing in the laundry room with my phone to my cheek, I'll call her and say, "Thank you. This is so important. I'm glad we can support our kids in respecting body boundaries together." I'll still be able to breathe as I say it. And she'll affirm, "I'm grateful to be parenting in community with you."

I will reach out to Meredith again fifteen years after I escaped, and she will say, "I always loved the healing that happened between us. And I continue finding women support each other so easily, and it's so necessary."

Violence has happened to my body. That will always be a fact. I still feel my vagina's scar. It aches some days how people say their knees can tell rain is coming. Other days, other hours, my vagina sings, not one song but many. Because healing has also happened to my body, between me and other bodies. Pleasure too. In a garden of more rooms, porches, text threads, changing tables, and moss couches than I can count, I have healed in the company of tenderness and love. I still do.

I've sometimes wondered: *Where does the healing work end and the regular old human work begin?* Now I see it's all the human work. The birthing, the tearing, the lovemaking, the scarring, the bleeding, the bathing, the listening, the singing, the feeding, the crying, the storytelling, the remembering, the discovering. I will never bounce back to who I was before I became a mother or to the girl I was before the abuse. I've stopped wanting that. I carry the past in my body, rivered with pains and repairs, but I also carry every possibility of the future, the love and pleasures seeking me. I'm here in my body, and I'm listening.

NOTES

Brennan, Madison. *Violations . . . And Then I Became Angry.* Jackson, MS: Lewis Art Gallery at Millsaps College, 2017.

Domonoske, Camila. "'Father of Gynecology,' Who Experimented on Slaves, No Longer on Pedestal in NYC." *NPR,* 2018. Accessed June 19, 2024. www.npr.org/sections/thetwo-way/2018/04/17/603163394/-father-of-gynecology-who-experimented-on-slaves-no-longer-on-pedestal-in-nyc.

Garza, Cristina Rivera. *Liliana's Invincible Summer: A Sister's Search for Justice.* New York: Hogarth, 2023.

Glück, Louise. "Nostos." In *Meadowlands.* New York: HarperCollins, 1997.

Heller, Marielle, dir. *A Beautiful Day in the Neighborhood.* 2019; Culver City, CA: TriStar Pictures, 2020. Film.

Jené, Sarah, and Jasmine Williams, in collaboration with Anna Burnett. *Moss Couch.* Jackson, MS: Mississippi Museum of Art, 2023.

Johnson, Kimberly Ann. *The Fourth Trimester: A Postpartum Guide to Healing Your Body, Balancing Your Emotions, & Restoring Your Vitality.* Boulder, CO: Shambhala, 2017.

Maltz, Wendy. *The Sexual Healing Journey: A Guide for Survivors of Sexual Abuse.* 3rd ed. New York: HarperCollins, 2012.

Michaels, Anne. *Fugitive Pieces.* New York: Random House, 1998.

Oppenheim, Maya. "Trump Administration 'Rolling Back Women's Rights by 50 years' by Changing Definitions of Domestic Violence and Sexual Assault" *The Independent*, 2019. Accessed June 19, 2024. www.independent.co.uk/news/world/americas/trump-domestic-abuse-sexual-assault-definition-womens-rights-justice-department-a8744546.html.

Perkins, Nichole, and Bim Adewunmi. "Thirst Aid Kit." Produced by *Slate*. Podcast. MP3 audio. https://slate.com/podcasts/thirst-aid-kit.

Rose, Jacqueline. *On Violence and On Violence Against Women.* New York: Farrar, Straus and Giroux, 2021.

Snyder, Rachel Louise. *No Visible Bruises: What We Don't Know About Domestic Violence Can Kill Us.* New York: Bloomsbury, 2019.

ACKNOWLEDGMENTS

The wisteria is at peak bloom as I write this. I must thank the land first, the unceded Choctaw land of Jackson, Mississippi. The animals, ground, and plants here gave me a path to write this story that was tolerable, moving me from dead, airless stories to new, oxygenated ones. Mississippi, you are my home.

To my agents, editors, and publishing team, my endless gratitude. Joelle Hann, you got the party started with the book proposal and dreamed big with me. You were by my side with so much heart and clarity as I became an author. *Viva la vida!* Claire Anderson-Wheeler, my first agent, your voice remained the tender and passionate editorial voice in my head as I wrote; your touch is everywhere in this book. Markus Hoffmann, you inspired trust at a crucial moment and took care of all the details. Shayna Keyles, my editor at North Atlantic Books, you believed that this book could be a powerful companion to women and to people in healing and you challenged me to get to the next layer in all the important places.

To the artists, musicians, and writers who kept me honest by the intimacy of their own work, especially Audre Lorde, Roxane Gay, Chanel Miller, Kiese Laymon, Raven Leilani, Ocean Vuong, Lidia Yuknavitch, Jesmyn Ward, Beth Ann Fennelly, and Molly Caro May. Special thanks to you. You reminded me it was worth trying, over and over, on days when the world was falling apart and my words on the page felt so small.

To the teachers, the sacred keepers, and the guides. I thank you with all my heart. To my entire birth and postpartum wellness teams. To my teachers Beth Graham, Priscilla Fermon, Anne MacMaster, and Kimberly Ann Johnson. To Dr. Hopkins for listening, believing, and helping me map my way to VITA NOVA; I'm telling everyone now. To my therapist Kristen for holding the tension of opposites with me.

To my friends and community, my gratitude abounds. You are too many to name; may it ever be so. Still I will name a few. For early reads and vital support: Christopher Guider, Molly Dunn, Eileen Rosete, and Colleen O'Mara-Diamond. For life-sustaining friendship and important conversations that got me through the times: Ruthie, Mary, Sophia, Meagan, Natalie, Matthew, Meredith, Alex, AmaJean, Morgan, LE, Amanda, and Andrew. To every person who has poured love into me and welcomed sharing uncomfortable truths within the safety and expansiveness of that love—you have made sharing this story possible.

To my family, my deepest thanks. For your fierceness, stories, and abundant love: Nana Jojo, Nana Grandma, Aunt Deborah. Thi-Dam Dong, the one photo we have of you traveled with me in my bag as I wrote. Mom, my light started with you, and your light stays with me always. Thank you for believing in the importance of my truthtelling. *Je t'aime.* Dad, thank you for taking me metal detecting to find the magic of the lost treasures; I love you through all the hard stories and am thankful for your presence in my life. Sally and Lloyd Sr., you welcomed me into your family in a more life-giving way than I could have imagined, and you have been champions of my writing. I am so grateful.

Acknowledgments

Lloyd, this is my story but it's also our story, and you trusted me with it completely. I will never forget how loved I felt by you as I wrote this book. How wide and free our love felt. How you encouraged every writing session and grew into your own beautiful expression of fatherhood in the process. To my children, Guider and Rowan, being by your side as you grow brings me abundant joy and wonder and inspires my most sacred intentions. Your presence in the world gave me the courage to use my voice in bolder ways than I ever had before, and I am forever changed by being your mother.

To my readers of *Unsilenced Woman*, I kept you close to my heart as I wrote this book. Because you opened your heart to my voice, I was able to open my heart and my voice even wider. Catherine Liggett, you are the embodiment of this. We heal together.

"Proud Flesh" first appeared in *The Audacity*, published by Roxane Gay in her Emerging Writer Series.

"The Skin Bridge" first appeared in the *Michigan Quarterly Review: Mixtape*.

ABOUT THE AUTHOR

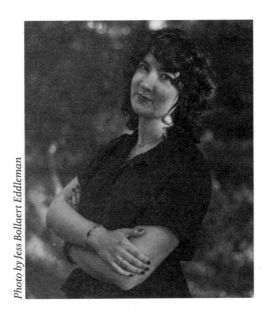

Catherine Simone Gray is a writer and educator. Her writings on motherhood and healing first appeared on her blog *Unsilenced Woman*. Featured by Roxane Gay in *The Audacity*'s Emerging Writer Series, her work has also appeared in *The Bitter Southerner* and the *Michigan Quarterly Review: Mixtape*. She is the recipient of a literary arts fellowship with the Mississippi Arts Commission. Catherine lives in Jackson, Mississippi, with her husband and their two sons.

ABOUT
NORTH ATLANTIC BOOKS

North Atlantic Books (NAB) is an independent, nonprofit publisher committed to a bold exploration of the relationships between mind, body, spirit, and nature. Founded in 1974, NAB aims to nurture a holistic view of the arts, sciences, humanities, and healing. To make a donation or to learn more about our books, authors, events, and newsletter, please visit www.northatlanticbooks.com.